Springer Series on Geriatric Nursing

Mathy D. Mezey, RN, EdD, FAAN, Series Editor
New York University Division of Nursing

Advisory Board: Margaret Dimond, PhD, RN, FAAN; Steven H. Ferris, Ph.D; Terry Fulmer, RN, PhD, FAAN; Linda Kaeser, PhD, RN, ACSW, FAAN; Virgene Kayser-Jones, PhD, RN, FAAN; Eugenia Siegler, MD; Neville E. Strumpf, PhD, RN, FAAN; May Wykle, PhD, RN, FAAN; Mary K. Walker, PhD, RN, FAAN

2004   **Restorative Care Nursing for Older Adults: A Guide for All Care Settings**
Barbara Resnick, PhD, CRNP, FAAN, FAANP

2004   **Care of Gastrointestinal Problems in the Older Adult**
Sue E. Meiner, EdD, APRN, BC, GNP

2003   **Geriatric Nursing Protocols for Best Practice, 2nd ed.**
Mathy D. Mezey, EdD, RN, FAAN, Terry Fulmer, PhD, RN, FAAN, Ivo Abraham
De Anne Zwicker, Managing Editor, MA, APRN, BC

2002   **Care of Arthritis in the Older Adult**
Ann Schmidt Luggen, PhD, RN, MSN, CS, BC-ARNP, and Sue E.

2002   **Prostate Cancer: Nursing Assessment, Management, and Care**
Meredith Wallace, PhD, RN, CS-ANP, and Lorrie L. Powel, PhD, RN

2002   **Bathing Without a Battle: Personal Care of Individuals With Dementia**
Ann Louise Barrick, PhD, Joanne Rader, RN, MN, FAAN, Beverly Hoeffer, DNSc, RN, FAAN,
and Phillip D. Sloane, MD, MPH

2001   **Critical Care Nursing of the Elderly, Second Edition**
Terry Fulmer, PhD, RN, FAAN, Marquis D. Foreman, PhD, RN, FAAN, Mary Walker, PhD, RN, FAAN, and
Kristen S. Montgomery, PhD, RNC, IBCLC

1999   **Geriatric Nursing Protocols for Best Practice**
Ivo Abraham, PhD, RN, FAAN, Melissa M. Bottrell, MPH, Terry T. Fulmer, PhD, RN, FAAN, and
Mathy D. Mezey, EdD, RN, FAAN

1998   **Home Care for Older Adults: A Guide for Families and Other Caregivers—Text and Instructor's Manual/Lesson Plan**
Mary Ann Rosswurm, EdD, RN, CS, FAAN

1998   **Restraint-Free Care: Individualized Approaches for Frail Elders**
Neville E. Strumpf, PhD, RN, C, FAAN, Joanne Patterson Robinson, PhD, RN, Joan Stockman Wagner, MSN,
CRNP, and Lois Evans, DNSc, RN, FAAN

1996   **Gerontology Review Guide for Nurses**
Elizabeth Chapman Shaid, RN, MSN, CRNP, and Kay Huber, DEd, RN, CRNP

1995   **Strengthening Geriatric Nursing Education**
Terry Fulmer, RN, PhD, FAAN, and Marianne Matzo, PhD, RN, CS

1994   **Nurse-Physician Collaboration: Care of Adults and the Elderly**
Eugenia L. Siegler, MD, and Fay W. Whitney, PhD, RN, FAAN

1993   **Health Assessment of the Older Individual, Second Edition**
Mathy D. Mezey, RN, EdD, FAAN, Louise H. Rauckhorst, RNC, ANP, EdD, and Shirlee Ann Stokes, RN, EdD, FAAN

1992   **Critical Care Nursing of the Elderly**
Terry T. Fulmer, RN, PhD, FAAN, and Mary K. Walker, PhD, RN, FAAN

About the Author

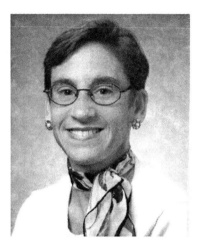

Barbara Resnick, PhD, CRNP, FAAN, FAANP holds a B.S.N. from the University of Connecticut, an M.S.N. from the University of Pennsylvania Gerontological Nurse Practitioner program, and a Ph.D. in Nursing from the University of Maryland. She maintains certification as a geriatric nurse practitioner from the American Nurses Credentialing Center. She is currently is an Associate Professor in the Department of Adult Health at the University of Maryland School of Nursing, and maintains a clinical/faculty position with clinical work at Roland Park Place, a Lifecare community. Dr. Resnick is a Fellow in the American Academy of Nurse Practitioners, and the American Academy of Nursing.

Dr. Resnick has over 100 articles published in nursing and/or medical journals, and numerous chapters in nursing textbooks related to care of the older adult. She has also presented on these topics nationally and internationally.

Dr. Resnick is currently on numerous Advisory Boards, including the Eastern Nursing Research Society, American Geriatrics Society, and Society of Behavioral Medicine. She is Chair of the Fellowship of the American Academy of Nurse Practitioners, Secretary of the American Academy of Nurse Practitioners 1996-2000, and Vice President Elect, President, and Past-President of the National Conference of Gerontological Nurse Practitioners 2001 to 2004. She serves on numerous other journal advisory boards such as Caring for the Ages, ElderHealth, Advance for Nurses, and the Internet Journal of Geriatrics and Gerontology.

Dr. Resnick also maintains an active clinical practice providing primary medical management to older adults in a variety of settings, and brings with her over 30 years of experience in long-term care. As a clinician she serves as a role model to other care providers working with older adults and strives to demonstrate innovative and exciting ways in which to motivate staff and older adults so that they can achieve their highest functional level, and maintain optimal health and quality of life.

Restorative Care Nursing for Older Adults

A Guide for All Care Settings

Barbara Resnick, *PhD, CRNP, FAAN, FAANP*
Associate Professor, Univerity of Maryland School of Nursing

Springer Publishing Company

This book is dedicated to: my four children, Aliza, Elie, Jacob, and Yael; my husband Howard; my mother Maidie Resnick; two brothers Frank and Yale; sister-in-laws Judy Resnick and Amy Sollins; and in-laws Helen and Leonard Sollins for their support, encouragement and patience with me; to all the older adults who have taught me about the challenges associated with aging and the ways in which they overcome those challenges; and lastly, to my father who taught me never to say "I can't."

Springer Publishing Company, Inc.
536 Broadway
New York, NY 10012-3955

Cover design by: Joanne Honigman
Acquisitions Editor: Ruth Chasek
Production Editor: Janice Stangel

01 02 03 04 05/5 4 3 2 1

Library of Congress Cataloging-in-Publication Data

Restorative care nursing for older adults : a guide for all care settings /
Barbara Resnick ... [et al.].
    p. ; cm. -- (Springer series on geriatric nursing)
  Includes bibliographical references and index.
  ISBN 0-8261-2454-2 (alk. paper)
  1. Geriatric nursing. 2. Rehabilitation nursing. 3. Older
people--Rehabilitation.
  [DNLM: 1. Rehabilitation Nursing--methods--Aged. 2.
Caregivers--education. 3. Recovery of Function--Aged. 4. Reimbursement
Mechanisms. WY 152 R4356 2004] I. Resnick, Barbara. II. Series.

RC954.R475 2004
618.97'0231--dc22   2004013002

Printed in the United States of America by Integrated Book Technology

Contents

List of Tables and Figures   vii

Contributors   ix

Preface   xi

1. Overview of Restorative Care   1
    Barbara Resnick and Robin E. Remsburg

2. Staff Education and Motivation: Establishing the Restorative Care Philosophy   13
    Barbara Resnick and Marjorie Simpson

3. Evaluating the Older Adult for Restorative Care   53
    Marianne Shaughnessy and Barbara Resnick

4. Restorative Care Activities   74
    Robin E. Remsburg

5. Motivating the Older Adult to Engage in Restorative Care   96
    Barbara Resnick

6. Documentation and Reimbursement for Restorative Care   112
    Annette Fleishell

    Appendix: The Interdisciplinary Team Approach   139
    Marjorie Simpson

Index   143

List of Tables and Figures

Table 1.1   Basic Goals of Restorative Care
Table 2.1   Overview of an Education Program for Restorative Care
Table 2.2   Components of Nursing Assistant Restorative Care Activities
Table 2.3   List of Weekly Classes for 6-Week Training Program
Table 2.4   Case Examples to Facilitate Discussion During Week One Inservice Training
Table 2.5   Incorporating Exercise Into Daily Activities
Table 2.6   Methods to Ensure Restorative Care Success
Table 2.7   Top 10 Reasons to Incorporate Restorative Care Into Daily Activities
Table 2.8   Examples of Long- and Short-Term Goals and Nursing Assistant Approaches
Table 2.9   Guidelines for Development of Goals
Figure 2.1   Power Point Presentations for Inservice Education
Table 3.1   Checklist for Restorative Care Evaluation
Table 3.2   List of Functional Scales
Table 3.3   Katz Index of ADLs
Table 3.4   Instrumental Activities of Daily Living
Table 3.5   Barthel Index
Table 3.6   Urinary Incontinence
Table 3.7   Differences in Signs and Symptoms Between Osteoarthritis and Rheumatoid Arthritis
Table 3.8   Evaluation of Falls
Table 3.9   Signs and Symptoms of Stroke
Table 3.10   Signs and Symptoms of Parkinson's Disease
Table 3.11   Characteristics of Dementia, Delirium, and Depression
Table 3.12   Typical and Atypical Signs and Symptoms of Depression
Table 3.13   Cognitive and Behavioral Measurement Tools
Table 3.14   Age-Related Changes in Sleep and the Sleep Cycle
Table 3.15   Contractures
Table 3.16   Muscle Strength Grading
Table 3.17   Steps for Doing Manual Muscle Testing
Table 3.18   Tool to Record Muscle Strength
Table 3.19   Gait Disorders
Table 3.20   Clock Drawing Scoring
Table 3.21   Exercise Definitions
Table 3.22   Need for Prescreening of Older Adults for Safe Exercise
Table 3.23   Warning Signs to Recognize During Exercise
Table 4.1   Goal Attainment Scales
Table 4.2   Assistive Devices for ADLs
Table 4.3   Components of ADLs

Table 4.4   Quality of Feeding Assistance Assessment
Table 4.5   Caregiver Behavior Checklist
Table 4.6   Recommendations for Grooming and Dressing Classes
Table 4.7   Exercise Program for Bedbound, Nonambulatory, and Ambulatory Older Adults
Table 4.8   Recommendations for Walking/Ambulation Groups
Table 4.9   Recommendations for Well-Attended Group Classes
Table 4.10   Group Classes Especially for Those with Cognitive Impairment
Table 5.1   Components of the Wheel of Motivation and Specific Interventions to Improve Motivation
Table 5.2   Age Changes Related to Motivation
Table 5.3   Normal Physiological Changes Associated With Aging
Table 5.4   Interventions to Improve Vision
Table 5.5   Interventions to Augment Hearing
Table 5.6   Strategies to Promote Independent Function in Cognitively Impaired Older Adults
Table 5.7   Verbal Encouragement Dos and Don'ts
Table 5.8   Identifying Unpleasant Sensations
Table 5.8a   Checklist for the Presence of Pain
Table 5.8b   Pain Assessment
Table 5.8c   Checklist for Evidence of Deconditioning
Table 5.9   Pursed Lip Breathing Exercises
Figure 5.1   Wheel of Motivation
Figure 5.2   Motivational Poster
Table 6.1   Activities of Daily Living as Defined by Federal Regulations
Table 6.2   Components of Restorative Care Nursing Programs
Table 6.3   MDS Requirements for Documentation and Assessment
Table 6.4   MDS Version 2.0 Special Treatment and Procedures
Table 6.5   MDS User's Manual Definitions of Functional Activities
Table 6.6   Restorative Care Flowsheet 1
Table 6.7   Restorative Care Flowsheet 2
Table 6.8   MDS Continence: Appliances and Programs
Table 6.9   Definition of Activities Under Scheduled Toileting and Bladder Retraining Programs
Table 6.10   CMS Criteria for Nursing Rehabilitation and Restorative Care
Table 6.11   Supportive Nursing Documentation for Therapies
Table 6.12   Suggestions for Documenting Resident's Inability to Participate in Treatment
Table 6.13   Restorative Care Resident Progress Note
Table 6.14   Restorative Care Resident Progress Note—Final Documentation
Table 6.15   Range of Motion Assessment and Initial Plan: Upper Extremity
Table 6.16   Range of Motion Assessment and Initial Plan: Lower Extremity
Table 6.17   Functional Assessment
Table 6.18   Federally Required Documentation of Restorative Care Activities
Table 6.19   Contractures Care Plan
Table 6.20   Definition and Requirements of the Care Plan
Table 6.21   Essential Components of Care Planning
Table 6.22   Resident Behavior Data-Gathering Tool
Table 6.23   Sample Documentation for Restorative Care Resident Class Attendance
Table 6.24   Documentation for Ambulation Class Attendance
Table 6.25   Restorative Care Program Quarterly Summary
Table 6.26   MDS Quality Indicators
Table 6.27   Clinical Links Among MDS-Based Quality Indicator Domains and Quality Indicators

Contributors

Marjorie Simpson, MS, CRNP, Doctoral Student
University of Maryland School of Nursing
Baltimore, MD

Marianne Shaughnessy, PhD, CRNP
Assistant Professor
University of Maryland School of Nursing
Baltimore, MD

Annette Fleishell, RN, BSN
Joanne Wilson's Gerontological Nursing Ventures
Laurel, MD

Robin Remsburg, PhD, APRN, BC
Johns Hopkins University School of Nursing
Baltimore, MD

Preface

Declining functional performance (e.g., in bathing, dressing, transferring, continence, ambulation, and stair climbing) has a great impact on older individuals and also on health care resources. For older adults across all care settings, loss of function alters the type and amount of nursing required, increases individuals risk of sequelae from immobility, and influences quality of life. Functional impairments have multifactorial causes and can be exacerbated by nursing care that creates dependency. In contrast, restorative care nursing focuses on the restoration and/or maintenance of physical function and helps older adults compensate for functional impairments and reach their highest level of function.

This book was written for caregivers (e.g., licensed nurses, nursing assistants, physical and occupational therapists, unpaid caregivers, social workers, and activities staff) and administrators at all levels of care to help them understand the basic philosophy of restorative care and to enable them to develop and implement successful restorative care programs. The book provides not only the material needed to educate caregivers about restorative care but, more importantly, educational material on ways to motivate older adults to engage in restorative care activities. In addition, the book provides an overview of the requirements for restorative care across all settings, discusses the necessary documentation, and provides tips for easily completing that documentation.

Acknowledgments

The information provided in this book is a reflection of over 20 years of work in the long term care environment. It pulls together the work of many individuals and I would like to acknowledge in particular the contributors to this wonderful resource. Over the years each of these individuals has endured my prodding to forever think out of the box and establish the innovative approaches to care of older adults in the long term care setting. In addition, I would like to thank the publishers who envisioned this as an important resource and supported our efforts. Most importantly, however, I would like to thank my family who forever endures the many hours that go into this type of work, and the older adults who are my teachers. What these individuals have shared regarding the benefits of physical activity and maintaining function, as well as the challenges associated with those activities, is at the core of this book

CHAPTER 1

Overview of Restorative Care

Barbara Resnick and Robin E. Remsburg

FUNCTIONAL PERFORMANCE OF OLDER ADULTS

The prevalence of persons needing assistance with activities of daily living (ADLs) in nursing homes, assisted living settings, and home care places significant burden on caregivers in these settings. Approximately 95% of current nursing home residents, 21% of assisted living facility residents, and 5%–13% of elderly community dwellers need assistance with one or more ADLs (Miller & Weissert, 2001).

Functional decline can result from injury, onset of new medical conditions, or worsening of preexisting chronic medical conditions. Functional decline can also occur gradually as a result of underuse. In long-term care settings residents' abilities to perform ADLs are influenced by the behaviors of caregivers in those settings (Barton, Baltes, & Orzech, 1980; Brubaker, 1996; Walk, Fleishman, & Mendelson, 1999; Winger & Schirm, 1989). Care patterns, such as providing too much assistance or an inappropriate type of assistance, can increase resident dependency. Excess disability, discrepancies between what individuals are able to do and what they actually perform are common in all care settings (Blair, 1996; Osborn & Marshall, 1993; Rogers, Holm, Burgio, Granieri et al., 1999; Rogers, Holm, Burgio, Hsu et al., 2000; Tappen, 1994). Both formal and informal caregivers can contribute to excess disability. A variety of factors, including a desire to be helpful, lack of knowledge and skill, and lack of time and staff, can result in increased dependency among impaired residents.

In general the type and amount of assistance nursing assistants provide to the institutionalized elderly promotes dependency (Blair, 1995; Kayser-Jones, 1997; Kayser-Jones & Schell, 1997a; Kayser-Jones & Schell, 1997b; Osborn & Marshal, 1993; Rogers et al., 1999; Tappen, 1994). Osborn and Marshall (1993) found that nursing home residents overwhelmingly were unassisted (did not receive help at all) or fully assisted (completely fed) by the nursing staff (both licensed and unlicensed) at mealtimes. Barton and colleagues (1980) found residents' dependent behaviors were supported by staff, while residents' independent self-care behaviors were ignored by staff. Brubaker (1996) found that whether the nurse performed ADL care or residents performed their own care was unpredictable and that for most residents nurse permission was needed to proceed with care activities.

Studies of interventions designed to improve ADL functioning demonstrate that functional decline can be stabilized or improved (Beck, Heacock, Mercer, Walls, Rapp, & Vogelpohl, 1997; Blair, 1999; Engleman, Mathews, & Altus, 2002; Remsburg, Armacost, Radu, & Bennett, 2001; Rogers et al., 1999; Schnelle, MacRae, Ouslander, Simmons, & Nitta, 1995; Tappen, 1994). Investigators hypothesize that residents' rapid response to behavioral interventions indicates alleviation of excess disabilities caused by care patterns rather than actual retraining and improvement in functional ability (Beck et al., 1997; Rogers et al., 1999; Tappen, 1994). Rogers and colleagues (1999), using a behavioral rehabilitation intervention with severely demented nursing home residents, demonstrated improved performance of morning care ADLs, with most residents responding within 5 days of the implementation. Over time, caregiving practices that promote dependency can result in increased impairment and disability and increased demands on caregivers. Providing appropriate ADL assistance, therefore, is critical in assisting impaired individuals to obtain and maintain optimal function.

ORIGIN AND DEFINITION OF RESTORATIVE CARE

Restorative care is driven by a need identified by observing residents living in long-term care settings. The majority of these individuals require some assistance with ADLs at the time of admission into the facilities (Aller & Coeling, 1995; National Investment Center, 1999). For institutionalized older adults, further loss of function alters the type and amount of nursing required, puts them at risk of sequelae from immobility, and influences quality of life (Challis et al., 2000; Kaplan, Strawbridge, Camacho, & Cohen, 1993; Mulrow, Gerety et al., 1994). It therefore became apparent to clinicians and policy makers that the focus of health care for older individuals should be to optimize function and comfort rather than to focus on the underlying disease process.

Many factors, however, influence the functional impairments noted in older individuals. These factors include lack of motivation (Mulrow, Chiodo et al., 1996; Resnick, 1998a), social issues and cultural expectations (Aller & Coeling, 1995; MaCrae et al., 1996), environmental factors (MaCrae et al., 1996), coexisting disease states (Ailinger, Dear, & Holley-Wilcox, 1993), and fear of falling (Hill, Schwarz, Kalogeropolulos, & Gibson, 1996). Nursing care, or care provided by family, friends, or significant others, that creates dependency (Davies, Ellis, & Laker, 2000; Resnick, 1998a; Waters, 1994) is a significant factor in promoting functional impairment in older adults. Unfortunately, caregivers often interpret changes in underlying ability as a sign of total helplessness and take on an increasing number of care activities, regardless of the individual's ability. This causes a progressive spiraling of loss for the individual, along with an ongoing decline in the individual's confidence in his or her ability to currently perform the task that has been subsumed by the nurse or caregiver. Further, caregivers tend to perform care-related activities in an attempt to increase manageability or because they feel it is the "caring" and humane thing to do.

Restorative nursing care takes an alternative approach to care by focusing on the restoration and/or maintenance of physical function and helping the older adult to compensate for functional impairments so that the highest level of function is obtained. The goal of this type of care is to maximize older adults' abilities by focusing on what the individuals *can do* versus what they can't do, optimizing independence, reducing the level of care required, and improving quality of life, self-image, and self-esteem.

Restorative care is not, however, the same as rehabilitation. Rehabilitation is defined as a continuing and comprehensive team effort to restore an individual to his or her former functional status or to maintain or maximize remaining function. Rehabilitation nursing is defined as the "diagnosis and treatment of human responses of individuals and groups to actual or potential health problems with the characteristics of altered functional ability and altered life-style" (Heffner, p. 27, 1995). Rehabilitation nurses generally have specialized knowledge and clinical skills to provide care for individuals with disabilities and to help families and significant others related to these individuals to cope with the disabilities. The goal of rehabilitation nursing is to assist the individual or group in the restoration and maintenance of maximum physical, psychosocial, and spirtual health. The nursing interventions generally are aimed to prevent complications of physical disability, restore optimal functioning, and help the individual adapt to an altered lifestyle. Moreover, rehabilitation is usually in response to an episodic event such as a stroke, hip fracture, or joint replacement. Goals are developed by the rehabilitation team and Medicare reimbursement is closely tied to achievement of those goals.

Conversely, restorative care is a philosophy of care which focuses on helping older adults to achieve and, more importantly, maintain optimal functional ability. The goals, unlike those of rehabilitation, are often focused on maintaining a specific function such as ambulating to the dining room or independent bathing and dressing (Table 1.1). Restorative care is a process of delivering minimal services that help maintain the highest possible level of function in older adult. In rehabilitation, services are allocated based on ability to achieve a reimbursable goal (e.g., being able to walk a functional distance). In contrast, all older adults have appropriate and relevant restorative care goals and should be exposed to restorative care services to achieve those goals. A chair- or bedbound resident

TABLE 1.1 Basic Goals of Restorative Care

Promote optimal mobility
Increase or maintain muscle strength and coordination
Promote continence
Prevent contractures
Promote independence in activities of daily living
Prevent pressure sores
Promote social activity
Provide a sense of accomplishment
Prevent isolation and depression
Improve motor skills
Improve communication
Provide opportunities for meaningful activities
Increase dignity and self-worth
Increase staff morale and job satisfaction

may benefit, for example, by participating in some strengthening activities, or simply by undergoing daily range of motion exercises to prevent contractures.

DESIGNATED RESTORATIVE CARE

Different models of restorative care have been described in the literature. The first model, referred to as the designated restorative care model, includes the development of specific restorative care programs and hiring and training designated nursing assistants or caregivers to perform the restorative care activities (Atkinson, 1992; Haffenreffer & Gold, 1991). Alternatively, restorative care nursing activities can be added to the current care provided to an older adult by any nurse, nursing assistant, or other caregiver (Orth, 1991). This type of model is referred to as an integrated restorative care program and is discussed in the following section. Finally, some settings implement specific restorative care programs such as a dining program, walk-to-dine program, or memory/communication program (Atkinson, 1992; Koroknay, Werner, Cohen-Mansfield, & Braun, 1995).

Designated restorative care programs have been used in long-term care settings (Remsburg, Armacost, Radu, & Bennett, 1999) as well as in home care (Tinetti et al., 2002). In these settings designated nurses and/or nursing assistants generally provide the restorative care interventions. Nurses or nursing assistants are trained on specific restorative care skills such as ambulating residents, implementing specific feeding techniques, or using assistive devices with residents to facilitate independent dressing. These programs may be affiliated with the rehabilitation department within a facility or home health agency, and referrals may be made to restorative care nursing when traditional rehabilitation services are completed. In designated programs, individuals generally receive restorative care services for a limited amount of time, for example, until a specific goal has been reached or maintained for a short period of time, until they refuse to participate, or until they are discharged from the facility. These designated restorative care services are generally scheduled at a time that is convenient for the nursing assistant or caregiver and must be implemented at that time. The nurse or nursing assistant providing these services will need to move on and begin working with another older individual.

One of the major problems in designated restorative care programs is that the older individual must perform any given restorative care activity at a time that is convenient for the nursing assistant or caregiver but may or may not be convenient for or preferred by the older individual. The designated caregiver has a rigid schedule for providing restorative care services. This might mean that an older adult has to perform bathing and dressing activities at a time when he or she is fatigued, in pain, or hungry. Clearly, caregiver-driven scheduling may not be the best way to facilitate the restorative care intervention.

Another major problem with a designated restorative care model is that once a decision is made to discontinue a restorative care service, the activity may not be assumed by other caregivers who have not been taught how to perform restorative care activities. For example Mrs. B, a resident in a long-term care facility, was referred from traditional physical therapy to restorative care with the goal of walking to the dining room for each meal. She was maintained on the restorative care program for 8 weeks, and the designated nursing assistant walked her daily to the dining room for each meal and provided the necessary encouragement and stand-by assistance. At the end of the 8-week period, it was decided that Mrs. B was stable and able to walk to the dining room and that, consequently, restorative care services would need to be discontinued. Unfortunately, what commonly occurs in such scenarios is that the resident is no longer encouraged to continue the activity. Mrs. B actually refused to ambulate with the regular staff. The nursing assistants working with her complained that it required too much time to encourage her to walk, and the other staff found it was easier to use a wheelchair and quickly facilitate the transport to the dining room.

INTEGRATED RESTORATIVE CARE PROGRAMS

In contrast to designated restorative care programs, integrated restorative care programs focus on implementing a pervasive philosophy of care geared toward helping all older adults obtain and maintain their optimal functional capability. This philosophy of care reinforces the individuals' underlying abilities and motivation to retain their highest level of independence. Integrated restorative care is an ongoing process that uses input from all disciplines to establish the best way to optimize an individual's underlying capability and functional performance. There is a commitment on the part of All staff are committed to promoting independent function, even though it may be quicker and easier for a nurse, nursing assistant, or other caregiver to perform the activity for the older adult. Restorative care activities are incorporated into daily activities and may be as simple as doing hand-over-hand bathing, using assistive devices to facilitate independent eating, or doing a daily exercise routine. These activities can be carried out during the course of the day by any nurse, nursing assistant, or caregiver working with that individual. Timing of the restorative care activity in an integrated model capitalizes on the individual's preference and personal schedule so that bathing, for example, is done when the older individual prefers. Ideally in integrated restorative care programs all nurses and nursing assistants will focus on function of the resident rather than task completion.

Integrated restorative care, therefore, occurs 24 hours a day, 7 days a week. During the course of the day and during all routine care activities, individuals should be encouraged to perform at their optimal functional level. In the long-term care setting or home, for example, if an older adult asks for a drink, the nurse, nursing assistant, or any person providing care should try to optimize function. The functional activity may vary depending on the individual's underlying capability. The nurse, nursing assistant, or caregiver might have the resident walk with him or her to obtain the drink or encourage the individual to get up and get a drink in the kitchen or pantry.

IMPLEMENTING A RESTORATIVE CARE PHILOSOPHY OF CARE

Understanding functional performance of older adults in any setting requires the consideration of multiple factors. Most importantly, the philosophy of care needs change from one that focuses on performing care activities for these individuals to a focus on the restoration and/or maintenance of physical function. While cure or complete restoration of function may not be realistic, most older adults can benefit from participation in a restorative care program, whether this benefit is psychological or physical (Bonn, 1999; Farnham & Moffett, 1988; Haffenreffer & Gold, 1991). Some individuals may benefit from having the increased social interaction that focuses on positive reinforcement of independent activities. Others may have a significant improvement in quality of life with increased independence (e.g., independent eating or improved continence). The burden of disability for caregivers may also be diminished by small improvements in older adults' performance of ADLs such as eating, dressing, or bathing. Ultimately this improvement can influence the cost of long-term care (Matsubayashi et al., 1998).

In 1987 the Omnibus Budget Reconciliation Act (OBRA) mandated that, for individuals living in long-term care settings, the facility must ensure that a resident's functional ability—based on a comprehensive assessment of the resident, particularly as related to ADLs—did not diminish unless circumstances of the individual's clinical condition demonstrated that the decline was unavoidable. Under the current reimbursement system, facilities are able to capture costs related to the provision of restorative care for their Medicare skilled residents if they document and demonstrate adherence to the required components of the program. These components include providing (1) two or more nursing rehabilitation activities for 15 or more minutes a day for 6 or more of the last 7 days and (2) nursing interventions that assist or promote the resident's ability to attain his or her maximum functional potential, promote the resident's ability to adapt and adjust to living as independently and safely as possible, and focus on optimal physical, mental, and psychosocial functioning. Restorative care activities do not include procedures or techniques carried out by qualified therapists.

PRIOR RESTORATIVE CARE RESEARCH

A recent study by Morris and colleagues (1999) provides some support for the utility of restorative care activities in nursing homes. This study tested a nursing rehabilitation program, that is, a restorative care program, and compared this against an exercise intervention, or routine care. The nursing rehabilitation program involved a five-step approach that evaluated the residents' ability to engage in functional activities and implemented interventions to encourage participation in personal care activities at residents' highest level of independence. Ten months after initiation of the program, individuals who received rehabilitation had less functional decline than those in the control group and the exercise intervention group.

Rogers and colleagues (1999) implemented an intervention that focused on helping cognitively impaired residents participate in morning care. This study demonstrated that with appropriate cues and nursing care, individuals with significant cognitive impairment could increase function with regard to morning care activities. Other studies (Evans, 1995; 1999; Fiatarone et al., 1994; Koroknay et al., 1995; Netz & Jacob, 1994; Paterson et al., 1999; Schnelle, MacRae et al., 1995; 1996; Schoenfelder, 2000) have demonstrated repeatedly that simple exercise interventions for older adults can have beneficial effects on maintaining function and improving overall quality of life.

Remsburg and colleagues (1999) compared two restorative care nursing programs: one that used designated nursing assistants (designated to provide restorative nursing care only) versus one that used integrated nursing assistants (i.e., those already working on the unit). The researchers found that, 6 months after starting the program, there was better enrollment, better staff documentation compliance for restorative care services, and greater staff satisfaction in the designated care program versus the integrated care program.

Tinnetti and colleagues (2002) studied the impact of a designated restorative care program in the home care setting. Specially trained home health staff, including nurses, nursing assistants, and physical and occupation therapists, developed and provided restorative care services to older adults in the home setting.

At the end of the exposure to restorative care services, the older individuals who received these services had better self-care scores, better home management skills, and better mobility when compared to individuals in the control group (i.e., those that received usual home care services). It is not clear, however, what happened to these individuals after the designated restorative care program was discontinued.

Although the studies (Remsburg et al., 1999; Tinnetti et al., 2002) supported a designated restorative care model, at least with regard to implementation, consideration must also be given to the fiscal and practical issues related to implementing and maintaining this type of program in all settings (Schnelle, Cruise, Rahman, & Ouslander, 1998). Obviously it is costly to hire staff to provide only restorative care services, particularly since these services are covered only for those who are eligible (see chapter 6). Using an integrated restorative care model is likely to be more realistic from the cost perspective. In addition, an integrated program allows for a more individualized approach in that the restorative care activities can be implemented any time during regular activities, not just when the restorative aide is scheduled to see the patient. The integrated approach also facilitates direct communication between the nurses, nursing assistants, and other caregivers and the physical, occupational, or speech therapists that may be involved with the individual and thereby helps all caregivers to carry over activities from traditional therapy to ongoing restorative care (Furnham & Moffet, 1988).

In response to the OBRA guidelines, managers in long-term care facilities have attempted to develop restorative care nursing programs to address the function and well-being of their residents. Manuals, such as *Stayin Alive: Developing and Implementing a Restorative Care Program* (Fleishell & Resnick, 1998) and *Restorative Nursing: A Training Manual for Nursing Assistants* (Tracey, 2000); videotapes (Resnick, 2001); and guidelines outlining the steps involved in developing these programs (Remsburg, Armacost et al., 1999; Resnick & Fleishell, 1999, 2002) have also been published. Although there have been some anecdotal and descriptive reports about these programs and their benefits (Farnham & Moffett, 1988; Koroknay et al., 1995; Orth, 1991; Resnick, Allen, & Ruane, 2002; Resnick & Fleischell, 1999), little work has been done to demonstrate the outcomes of these programs. Moreover, the studies done previously (Morris et al., 1999; Remsburg,

Luking et al., 2001; Resnick, Allen, & Ruane, 2002) did not focus on changing behavior in nursing assistants and residents. Motivating nursing assistants and residents to engage in restorative care activities and teaching and reinforcing a new philosophy of care that focuses on function are both essential to successful restorative care programs. Although restorative care has not yet been tested in a randomized, controlled setting, the Agency for Health, Research, and Quality (AHRQ) recently funded a large multisite study to test an integrated restorative care program specifically designed to change the behavior of both care providers and older individuals over time (Resnick, 2002).

LEADERSHIP ROLE IN IMPLEMENTATION OF A RESTORATIVE CARE PHILOSOPHY

As previously described, there are different models of restorative care, none of which have been systematically evaluated for effectiveness through randomized, controlled trials. The 1987 OBRA guidelines mandate that long-term care facilities demonstrate that function is optimally maintained in residents, and there is increased interest by clinicians and policy makers to focus on function in all care settings. Unfortunately, as yet there are no specific components of what should be included in a successful restorative care program, and/or how to implement such programs. Some guidelines, however, can be used from behavior change research and implementation of other types of programs in a variety of settings. The role of leadership is particularly important, as is utilization of appropriate techniques to educate and motivate both caregivers and older adults.

Implementation of a restorative care philosophy requires understanding and support from the formal and informal leadership within the setting. Leaders in these settings should be willing to set an appropriate example for all other who provide care for or interact with the older individual. Leaders must, for example, demonstrate a restorative care philosophy at all times. In addition, the leaders in any care setting should clarify the expectations of the caregivers who will interact with the older individual and provide the necessary resources so that appropriate training can be done. These leaders will need to provide appropriate feedback to the caregivers in these settings and encourage ongoing implementation of the restorative care activities.

The formal leadership within any setting includes key individuals who are involved with identifying and implementing ways to meet the organization's goals and objectives. Key formal leadership positions in the long-term care setting include administrator, director of nursing, and medical director. The informal leadership includes individuals who, by virtue of skill, attitude, or longevity, tend to influence the attitudes and performance of others within the facility. In home care settings there are likely to be administrative support staff; a director of nursing and medical care; speech, occupational, and physical therapy personnel; and other leaders.

The leadership's commitment to the restorative care program will influence the staff's enthusiasm and dedication. The formal facility leadership should identify and agree on the value of implementing a restorative care philosophy within the facility. Ethical concerns, for example, should be considered, and the administration needs to support staff as they encourage older individuals to engage in self-care. If, for example, the administration sides with a family member who is upset that the nursing assistant is "making Mom walk to the dining room," this would contradict any stated support of a restorative care philosophy.

Once a decision has been made to implement a restorative care philosophy, leaders need to be involved with developing the list of functions and tasks necessary for the implementation process to succeed. A task force of appropriate individuals (e.g., nursing home administrator, medical director, director of nursing, social worker, advanced practice nurse, and physical, occupational, and speech therapists) can be very useful in developing the list of functions and establishing who is most appropriate to do what. Having leadership involved in this process will provide the necessary framework for other staff and caregivers to proceed and will ensure that resources are allocated for all tasks to be completed.

TRAINING FOR RESTORATIVE CARE ACTIVITIES: USING A SELF-EFFICACY FRAMEWORK

A major focus of implementing a restorative care program is on changing the behavior of care providers who interact with the older individual so that the focus of care is on function and maintenance of function rather than on getting care needs met. Employee training approaches traditionally provide information for the employee to perform the tasks required in the job description. Using the self-efficacy framework (Bandura, 1977), however, is an effective way to enhance a job-training program. The self-efficacy framework conceptualizes motivation within the broader spectrum of social cognitive theory and the theory of self-efficacy. Social cognitive theory is based on triadic reciprocity, suggesting that behavior, cognitive, other personal factors, and environmental influences all operate interactively as determinants of each other. There is mutual action between causal factors, and behavior can be manipulated by these interactions. Bandura (1977; 1986; 1995; 1997) specifically suggested that efficacy expectations were critical to motivation. These efficacy expectations include self-efficacy, which is an individual's judgment of his or her abilities to organize and execute courses of action to accomplish specific goals, and outcome expectancy, which is the belief that performing a specific behavior will result in a certain outcome.

Efficacy expectations are dynamic and are both appraised and enhanced by four mechanisms (Bandura, 1997): (1) enactive mastery experience, or successful performance of the activity of interest; (2) verbal persuasion, or verbal encouragement given by a credible source that the individual is capable of performing the activity of interest; (3) vicarious experience, or seeing like individuals perform a specific activity; and (4) physiological and affective states such as pain, fatigue, or anxiety associated with a given activity. The theory of self-efficacy suggests that the stronger the individual's efficacy expectations (self-efficacy and outcome expectations), the more likely he or she will be to initiate and persist with a given activity.

In a study by Wolfe, Nordstrom, and Williams (1998), which tested the impact of a pre-employment telemarketing-training program on self-efficacy, the group that received the intervention had stronger self-efficacy expectations related to job performance and remained employed significantly longer than the control group. Studies that use self-efficacy to predict job performance have subsequently begun to emerge. Employees with high self-efficacy more effectively seek and use feedback obtained from managers and peers to improve their role clarity and job performance (Brown, Ganesan, & Challagalla, 2001). Additionally, employees with higher self-efficacy have lower job-related stressor strain and demonstrate more effective

coping styles than employees with lower levels of self-efficacy (Jex, Bliese, Buzzell, & Primeau, 2001). Building self-efficacy, therefore, related to performance of restorative care activities for nursing assistants, can potentially not only help job performance, but also improve retention.

TRAINING INTERVENTIONS TO INFLUENCE BEHAVIOR OF NURSING ASSISTANTS

Several interventions have been implemented to change behavior of nursing assistants and teach them to encourage increased resident participation in ADLs. Beck and colleagues (Beck, Heacock, Rapp, & Mercer, 1993; Beck, Heacock, Mercer et al., 1995) tested Strategies to Promote Independence in Dressing (SPID), which is a training program that matches the residents' needed level of assistance with their underlying ability and provides some additional training for nursing assistants on how to facilitate performance of ADLs. The program includes motivation of the resident and provides immediate reinforcers for successfully performing a dressing task (Vogelpohl, Beck, Heacock, & Mercer, 1996).

Blair (1996) developed and tested an intervention to encourage independence in functional activities using mutual goal setting and behavioral procedures focusing on prompting, shaping, and providing reinforcement to get older adults to engage in functional activities. Goal setting had a positive effect on the older adults' self-care activities, and positive reinforcement was effective in motivating these residents to perform self-care activities. Similarly, Morris and colleagues (1999) developed and tested an intervention, "Self Care for Seniors" that incorporates five steps, which include evaluating the older adult's ability, developing appropriate goals and a plan of care based on those abilities, and selecting environmental, communication, and motivational guidelines that assist the older adult in self-care activities. In addition, an intervention that focused on training nursing assistants to increase communication with older individuals had a positive effect on function, behavior, and social isolation (Allen-Burge, Stevens, & Burgio, 1999; Burgio & Stevens, 1999).

These studies all demonstrate that caregiver interactions with older adults that incorporate careful evaluation of individuals' underlying ability, goal setting, and positive verbal encouragement can improve the functional performance of those individuals. None of the studies considered the outcome expectations of either the nursing assistants or the older adults involved with regard to restorative care activities. In these studies, there was no consideration given to the beliefs of either the caregivers or the older individuals related to performance of restorative care activities. Did the older individuals and/or caregivers believe that performing restorative care activities would help the older individual get stronger, feel better, or have a better quality of life? Did they believe that it was dangerous to encourage performance of restorative care activities because the older adult might hurt a joint or pull a muscle? Did the caregivers believe that restorative care would mean more work for them and thereby increase their anxiety about completing a full assignment of patient care?

There were also concerns about treatment fidelity in some of the studies described above because no consideration was given to the transference of new skills into the everyday clinical practice of the nursing assistants (Blair, 1996; Morris et al., 1999). Consequently it is not clear how closely the interventions were adhered to in these studies. Other researchers who studied interventions that focus on changing care behaviors (Remsburg Palmer, Langford, & Mendelson, 1999; Schnelle, Cruise, Rahman, & Ouslander, 1998) found that care providers exposed to these interventions usually reverted back to preintervention behavior that continued to encourage dependency.

BARRIERS TO IMPLEMENTING RESTORATIVE CARE

Barriers to implementing restorative care can arise from the older individual or from the caregiver. Resident-related barriers include medical conditions such as pain and depression, disease and age-related conditions such as dementia and sensory decline, resident and family misconceptions about aging and functional abilities, resident and family expectations of caregivers, deconditioning, embarrassment, fear of injury or failure, and transient conditions such as fatigue, discomfort from unmet toileting needs, and medication side effects such as nausea (Cumming, Salkeld, Thomas, & Szonyi, 2000; Marx, Werner, Cohen-Mansfield, & Feldman, 1992; Means, Currie, & Gershkoff, 1993; Resnick, 2000; Schultz, Ellingrod, Tuevey, Moser, & Arndt, 2003; Wu, 2002). Before initiating restorative care, medical conditions affecting functional performance should be addressed. Analgesia for painful conditions such as osteoarthritis should be administered. Residents should be routinely assessed for signs of depression and treated if needed. Residents and families often have misconceptions about older persons' self-care abilities. Older adults and their families who expect caregiving staff to perform ADL tasks rather than assist the older adult to perform tasks may need education on the benefits and goals of restorative care.

Caregiving staff barriers to providing restorative care include lack of time, lack of knowledge and training, inadequate support and recognition, lack of planning and organization, lack of resources, and lack of perceived benefit (Crogan & Shultz, 2000; Smith, 1998, Lekan-Rutledge, Palmer, & Belyea, M, 1998; Schnelle, Kapur et al., 2003). A major excuse for dependency-promoting care is staff time (Blair, 1995). Studies of restorative interventions have demonstrated that caregivers can learn and implement restorative techniques that improve older adults' self-care abilities (Blair, 1995). Unfortunately when study interventions end, caregivers often revert back to prestudy caregiving patterns (Blair, 1995; Colling, Ouslander, Hadley, Eisch, & Campbell, 1992; Schnelle, 1990). Restorative care activities can be incorporated into regular care and therefore should not take a significant amount of time to complete (Beck, Heacock, Mercer et al., 1995; Lange-Alberts & Shott, 1994; Schnelle, MacRae et al., 1995; Simmons, Osterweil, Schnelle, 2001). Beck, Heacock, Mercer, and colleagues (1995) demonstrated a time increase of only 1 minute for a self-dressing intervention with cognitively impaired residents, and Schnelle and colleagues demonstrated only a 2-minute increase in time needed to assist residents with prompted voiding compared to changing a soiled incontinence pad. Lange-Alberts and Shott (1994) found improvements in calorie consumption with a 5-minute cueing and prompting intervention.

Strengthening the self-efficacy and outcome expectations of care providers can help increase motivation and eliminate some of these barriers to continuing restorative care activities. The five-step approach described below focuses on changing behavior in both nursing assistants and older adults by strengthening self-efficacy and outcome expectations. Ultimately this will lead to an enduring change in the philosophy of care provided to older adults and facilitate a focus on function through restorative care.

THE FIVE-STEP APPROACH

In the five-step approach to implementing a restorative care program, interventions are used to strengthen self-efficacy and outcome expectations relate to restorative care activities of the nurses, nursing assistants, and other caregivers. The approach provides the tools to motivate older individuals to likewise engage in restorative care activities. Initially, the goal of the five-step approach is to educate and train caregivers in restorative care activities, and then the caregivers need to use what they learned to motivate older adults to participate in restorative care activities. The specific steps include (1) establishing an appropriate philosophy of care, which involves educating and motivating staff; (2) evaluating the older adult; (3) establishing a routine of restorative care activities; (4) motivating the older adult to engage in functional activities; and (5) documentation, reevaluation, and demonstrating outcomes. These five steps will provide an organizing framework for this book.

RESTORATIVE CARE IN ANY SETTING

Although restorative care and restorative care programs have generally been associated with long-term care settings, a restorative care philosophy is appropriate and indicated for every setting that provides services to older adults. Assisted living is a state-regulated and -monitored residential long-term care option. Assisted living provides or coordinates oversight and services to meet the individualized needs of each older adult based on a comprehensive assessment of his or her underlying functional ability and performance. The ultimate goal of these services is to promote dignity, autonomy, independence, and quality of life (Assisted Living Workgroup, 2003). While there are currently no federal guidelines to require this type of care consistently across all states, assisted living settings are geared to helping older adults remain in those settings for life. Clearly, a restorative care philosophy is necessary to achieve optimal maintenance of function

and allow the older adults to remain in this type of care setting. The current recommendations to the United States Senate developed by the Assisted Living Workgroup (2003) are currently under review. These recommendations, however, suggest that function be optimized and maintained by promoting and encouraging self-care and exercise.

Home health care is also now mandated to focus on function. The Medicare home health care program moved to a prospective payment system on October 1, 2000. Now consistent with acute care and long-term care settings, reimbursement to home health is not based on the actual cost of care and services. Instead the agency is provided with a predetermined amount based on clinical indicators identified from the documented Outcome and Assessment Information Set (OASIS). The OASIS is a group of data elements that represent core items of a comprehensive assessment for an older adult in the home setting and includes basic information about the individual, environmental factors, social factors, and ability to perform ADLs such as bathing and dressing and instrumental activities of daily living including managing finances and taking medications. With the outcomes-based payment limitation, the care planning focus must be on helping patients to quickly obtain and maintain their overall health and function. In order to do this, Marrelli (2003) strongly recommends borrowing the restorative care philosophy from the long-term care setting. The focus again would be on helping older adults to meet and maintain their highest functional level.

Unfortunately, no matter the setting in which the older adult lives, there are common discrepancies between what the individual is able to do (i.e., can do) versus what he or she actually does (i.e., performance). Bootsma-van der Wiel and colleagues (2001) studied 599 older adults (age 85 and above) living in the community and noted that the prevalence of disability, defined as inability to perform one or more ADL, was 64% for women and 55% for men. The prevalence of disability defined as inactivity (i.e., not performing despite underlying ability) was 92% for women and 98% for men. There was a significant discrepancy between what these individuals were able to do and what they actually performed. Similarly, there are discrepancies between underlying ability and actual performance of functional activities in the long-term care setting and assisted living (Resnick, 1999; Resnick & Bellantonio, 2003). Residents have admitted that they are capable of doing their own bathing and dressing but because the nurse comes in and completes the task for them, they simply do not do it.

Restorative care can and should be implemented in any setting in which older adults are living. The subsequent chapters in this book provide the tools and techniques needed to implement this type of care philosophy in all settings. What may vary are the resources available to implement these techniques and the ability to control the setting in which care activities are occurring. In the home setting, for example, there may or may not be a caregiver routinely. The older adult may be resourceful and recruit someone to complete a task as it is needed. This person could be a well-meaning neighbor, friend, or relative. Certainly it is harder to control and correct these types of interactions. In assisted living or long-term care settings, care providers are more accessible and therefore may take over care activities that the individual can do alone. The challenge is trying to reach, educate, and support the appropriate caregivers. In addition, no restorative care program is complete without working with older adults to help them understand and believe in the benefits of restorative care.

REFERENCES

Ailinger, R., Dear, M., & Holley-Wilcox, P. (1993). Predictors of function among older Hispanic immigrants: A five-year follow-up. *Nursing Research, 42*(4), 240–244.

Allen-Burge R., Stevens, A.B., & Burgio L.D. (1999). Effective behavioral interventions for decreasing dementia-related challenging behavior in nursing homes. *International Journal of Geriatric Psychiatry, 14*(3), 213–228; discussion 228–232.

Aller, L., & Coeling, H. (1995). Quality of life: Its meaning to the long-term care resident. *Journal of Gerontological Nursing, 21*(2), 20–25.

Atkinson, D. (1992). Restorative nursing: A concept whose time has come. *Nursing Homes, 4*(1), 9–12.

Bandura, A. (1997). *Self-efficacy: The exercise of control.* New York: W.H. Freeman and Company.

Barton, E.M., Baltes, M.M., & Orzech, M.J. (1980). Etiology of dependence in older nursing home residents during morning care: the role of staff behavior. *J Per Soc Psychol, 38*(3), 423–431.

Beck, C., Heacock, P., Rapp, C., & Mercer, S. (1993). Assisting cognitively impaired elders with activities of daily living. *American Journal of Alzheimer's Care and Related Disorders and Research, 8*(6), 11–20.

Beck, C., Ortigara, A., Mercer, S., & Shue, V. (1999). Enabling and empowering certified nursing assistants for quality dementia care. *International Journal of Geriatric Psychiatry, 14*(3), 197–211.

Blair, C.E. (1995). Combining behavior management and mutual goal setting to reduce physical dependency in nursing home residents. *Nursing Research, 44*(3), 160–165.

Blair, C. (1996). Combining behavior management and mutual goal setting to reduce physical dependency in nursing home residents. *Nursing Research, 44*(3), 160–164.

Bootsma-van der Wiel, A., Gussekloo, J., De Craen, A., Van Exel, E., Knook, D., Lagaay, A., & Westendorp, R. (2001). Disability in the oldest old: "Can Do" or "Do Do"? *Journal of the American Geriatrics Society, 49,* 909–914.

Bonn, K. (1999). Resuming restorative care. *Nursing Homes, 6,* 72.

Brown, S., Ganesan, S., & Challagalla, G. (2001). Self-efficacy as a moderator of information-seeking effectiveness. *Journal of Applied Psychology, 86*(5), 1043–1051.

Brubaker, B.H. (1996). Self-care in nursing home residents. *Journal of Gerontological Nursing, 22*(7), 22–30.

Challis, D., Mozley, C.G., Sutcliffe, C., Bagley, H., Price, L., Burns, A., Huxley, P., & Cordingley, L. (2000). Dependency in older people recently admitted to care homes. *Age and Ageing, 29,* 255–260.

Colling, J., Ouslander, J., Hadley, B.J., Eisch, J., & Campbell, E. (1992). The effects of patterned urge-response toileting (PURT) on urinary incontinence among nursing home residents. *Journal of the American Geriatric Society, 40*(2), 135–141.

Cumming, R.G., Salkeld, G., Thomas, M., & Szonyi, G. (2000). Prospective study of the impact of fear of falling on activities of daily living, SF–36 scores, and nursing home admission. *Journal of Gerontology Series A Biological Sciences Medicine and Science, 55*(5), M299–M305.

Crogan, N.L., & Shultz, J.A. (2000). Nursing assistants' perceptions of barriers to nutrition care for residents in long-term care facilities. *Journal of Nurses Staff Development, 16*(5), 216–221.

Davies, S., Ellis, L., & Laker, S. (2000). Promoting autonomy and independence for older people within nursing practice: An observational study. *Journal of Clinical Nursing, 9,* 127–136.

Evans, W. (1995). Effects of exercise on body composition and functional capacity of the elderly. *Journal of Gerontology A Biological Sciences Medicine and Science, 50,* 147–150.

Farnham, N., & Moffett, J. (1988). Coordinated rehabilitation exercise improves quality. *Provider, 14*(9), 39.

Fiatarone, M., O'Neill, E., Ryan, N., Clements, K., Solares, G., Nelson, M., Roberts, S., Kehayias, J., Lipsitz, L., &

Evans, W. (1994). Exercise training and nutritional supplementation for physical frailty in very elderly people. *The New England Journal of Medicine, 330*(25), 1721–1727.

Fleishell, A., & Resnick, B. (1998). *Stayin alive: Developing and implementing a restorative care nursing program*. Handbook developed by Joanne Wilson's Gerontological Nursing Ventures, Laurel, Maryland.

Haffenreffer, D., & Gold, M.F. (1991). The rewards of restorative care. *Provider, 12,* 15–21.

Heffner, M. (1995). Lessons in courage. *Journal of Christian Nursing, 12*(4), 47–48.

Hill, K., Schwarz, J., Kalogeropololulos, A., & Gibson, S. (1996). Fear of falling revisited. *Archives of Physical Medicine and Rehabilitation, 77,* 1025–1029.

Jex, S., Bliese, P., Buzzell, S., & Primeau, J. (2001). The impact of self-efficacy on stressor-strain relations: Coping style as an explanatory mechanism. *Journal of Applied Psychology, 86*(3), 401–409.

Kaplan, G., Strawbridge, W., Camacho, T., & Cohen, R. (1993). Factors associated with change in physical functioning in the elderly. *Journal of Aging and Health, 5,* 140–153.

Kayser-Jones J. (1997). Inadequate staffing at mealtime. Implications for nursing and health policy. *Journal of Gerontological Nursing, 23*(8), 14–21.

Kayser-Jones, J., & Schell, E. (1997a). The effect of staffing on the quality of care at mealtime. *Nursing Outlook, 45*(2), 64–72.

Kayser-Jones, J., & Schell, E. (1997b). The mealtime experience of a cognitively impaired elder: Ineffective and effective strategies. *Journal of Gerontological Nursing, 23*(7), 33–39.

Koroknay, V., Werner, P., Cohen-Mansfield, J., & Braun, J. (1995). Maintaining ambulation in the frail nursing home resident: A nursing administered walking program. *Journal of Gerontological Nursing, 21*(11), 18–24.

Lange-Alberts, M.E., & Shott, S. (1994). Nutritional intake. Use of touch and verbal cuing. *Journal of Gerontological Nursing, 20*(2), 36–40.

Lekan-Rutledge, D., Palmer, M.H., & Belyea, M. (1998). In their own words: Nursing assistants' perceptions of barriers to implementation of prompted voiding in long-term care. *The Gerontologist, 38*(3), 370–378.

MaCrae, P., Asplund, L., Schnelle, J., Ouslander, J., Abrahamse, A., & Morris, C. (1996). A walking program for nursing home residents: Effects on walk endurance, physical activity, mobility and quality of life. *Journal of the American Geriatrics Society, 44,* 175–180.

Marrelli, T.M. (2003). Restorative care and home care: New implications for aide and nurse roles? *Geriatric Nursing, 24*(2), 128–129.

Marx, M.S., Werner, P., Cohen-Mansfield, J., & Feldman, R. (1992). The relationship between low vision and performance of activities of daily living in nursing home residents. *Journal of the American Geriatrics Society, 40*(10), 1018–1020.

Matsubayashi, K., Okumiya, K., Wada, T., Osaki, Y., Fujisawa, M., Doi, Y., & Ozawa, T. (1998). Improvement in self-care may lower the increasing rate of medical expenses for community-dwelling older people in Japan. *Journal of the American Geriatrics Society, 46*(11), 1484–1485.

Means, K.M., Currie, D.M., & Gershkoff, A.M. (1993). Geriatric rehabilitation. 4. Assessment, preservation, and enhancement of fitness and function. *Archives of Physical Medicine and Rehabilitation, 74*(5-S), S417–S420.

Miller, E.A., & Weissert, W.G. (2000). Predicting elderly people's risk for nursing home placement, hospitalization, functional impairment, and mortality: A synthesis. *Medical Care Research Review, 57*(3), 259–297.

Miller, E.A., Weissert, W.G. (2001). Incidence of four adverse outcomes in the elderly population: implications for home care policy and research, *Home Health Care Serv Q, 20*(4), 14–47.

Morris, J.N., Fiatarone, M., Kiely, D.K., Belleville-Taylor, P., Murphy, K., Littehale, S., Ooi, W.L., O'Neill, E., & Doyle, N. (1999). Nursing rehabilitation and exercise strategies in the nursing home. *Journal of Gerontology Series A Medical Sciences, 54A,* M494–M500.

Mulrow, C., Chiodo, L., Gerety, M., Lee, S., Basu, S., & Nelson, D. (1996). Function and medical comorbidity in south Texas nursing home residents: Variations by ethnic group. *Journal of the American Geriatrics Society, 44,* 279–284.

Mulrow, C., Gerety, M., Kanten, D., Cornell, J., Denino, L., Chiodo, L., Aguilar, C., O'Neil, M., Rosenberg, J., & Solis, R. (1994). A randomized trial of physical rehabilitation for very frail nursing home residents. *Journal of the American Medical Association, 271*(7), 519–524.

National Investment Center. (1999). Available on the Web site: http://www.nicinfo.org.

Netz, Y., & Jacob, T. (1994). Exercise and the psychological state of institutuionalized elderly: A review. *Perceptual Motor Skills, 79,* 1107–1118.

Orth, R. (1991). Restorative dining promotes independence, self-esteem. *Provider, 17*(12), 33.

Osborn, C.L., & Marshall, M.J. (1993). Self-feeding performance in nursing home residents. *Journal of Gerontological Nursing, 19*(3), 7–14.

Remsburg, R., Armacost, K., Radu, C., & Bennett, R. (1999). Two models of restorative nursing care in the nursing home: Designated versus integrated restorative nursing assistants. *Geriatric Nursing, 20,* 321–326.

Remsburg, R.E., Luking, A., Baran, P., Radu, C., Pineda,

D., Bennett, R.G., & Tayback, M. (2001). Impact of a comprehensive dining intervention, on weight and biochemical indicators of nutritional status—A pilot study. *Journal of the American Dietetic Association, 101*(12), 1460–1463.

Remsburg, R., Palmer, M.H., Langford, A.M., & Mendelson, G. (1999). Staff compliance with and ratings of effectiveness of a prompted voiding program in a long-term care facility. *Journal of Wound Ostomy Continence Nursing, 26*(5), 261–269.

Resnick, B. (1998a). Motivating the older adult to perform functional activites. *Journal of Gerontological Nursing, 24,* 23–31.

Resnick, B. (1999). Motivation in the older adult: Can a leopard change its spots? *Journal of Advanced Nursing, 29,* 792–799.

Resnick, B. (2000). Functional performance and exercise of older adults in long term care. *Journal of Gerontological Nursing, 26*(3), 7–16.

Resnick, B. (2001). Video Press, Inc. Developed a series of 5 tapes on Restorative care and motivating older adults to engage in these activities, Baltimore, MD, 2001. Available online at videopress.org.

Resnick, B., Allen, P., & Ruane, K. (2002). Testing the effectiveness of a restorative care program. *Long-Term Care Interface, 3*(11), 25–30.

Resnick, B., & Bellantunio, S. (2003). Research in Assisted Living Settings. *American Medical Directors Association meeting.* Orlando, Florida, March 2003.

Resnick, B., & Fleishell, A. (1998). *Stayin alive: Developing and implementing a restorative care program.* Training Manual. Laurel, MD: Joanne Wilson's Gerontological Nursing Ventures.

Resnick, B., & Fleishell, A. (1999). Restoring quality of life. *Advance for Nurses, 1,* 10–12.

Resnick, B., & Fleishell, A. (2002). Developing and implementing a successful restorative care program. *American Journal of Nursing, 102*(7), 91–95.

Rogers, J., Holm, M., Burgio, L., Granieri, E., Hsu, C., Hardin, J., & McDowell, B. (1999). Improving morning care routines of nursing home residents with dementia. *Journal of the American Geriatrics Society, 47*(9), 1049–1057

Rogers, J.C., Holm, M.B., Burgio, L.D., Hsu, C., Hardin, J.M., & McDowell, B.J. (2000). Excess disability during morning care in nursing home residents with dementia. *International Psychogeriatrics, 12*(2), 267–282.

Schnelle, J.F. (1990). Treatment of urinary incontinence in nursing home patients by prompted voiding. *J Am Geriatr Soc, 38*(3), 356–360.

Schnelle, J., Cruise, P., Rahman, A., & Ouslander, J. (1998). Developing rehabilitative behavioral interventions for long-term care: Technology transfer, acceptance and maintenance issues. *Journal of the American Geriatrics Society, 46,* 771–777.

Schnelle, J.F., Kapur, K., Alessi, C., Osterweil, D., Beck, J.G., Al-Samarrai, N.R., & Ouslander, J.G. (2003). Does an exercise and incontinence intervention save healthcare costs in a nursing home population? *Journal of the American Geriatrics Society, 51*(2), 161–168.

Schnelle J., MacRae, P., Ouslander, J., Simmons, S., & Nitta, M. (1995). Functional incidental training, mobility performance and incontinence care with nursing home residents. *Journal of the American Geriatrics Society, 43,* 1356–1362.

Schoenfelder, D. (2000). A fall prevention program for elderly individuals. Exercise in nursing homes. *Journal of Gerontological Nursing, 26*(3), 43–51.

Schultz, S.K., Ellingrod, V.L., Turvey, C., Moser, D.J., & Arndt, S. (2003). The influence of cognitive impairment and behavioral dysregulation on daily functioning in the nursing home setting. *American Journal of Psychiatry, 160*(3), 582–584.

Simmons, S.F., Osterweil, D., & Schnelle, J.F. (2001). Improving food intake in nursing home residents with feeding assistance: A staffing analysis. *Journal of Gerontology Series A Biological Sciences Medicine and Science, 56*(12), M790–M794.

Tappen, R.M. (1994). The effect of skill training on functional abilities of nursing home residents with dementia. *Research in Nursing and Health, 17*(3), 159–165.

Tinetti, M. (1986). Performance oriented assessment of mobility problems in elderly patients. *Journal of the American Geriatric Society, 34,* 199–206.

Tinetti, M.E., Baker, D., Gallo, W.T., Nanda, A., Charpentier, P., & O'Leary, J. (2002). Evaluation of restorative care vs usual care for older adults receiving an acute episode of home care. *Journal of the American Medical Association, 287*(16), 2098–2105.

Tracey, C. (2000). *Restorative nursing: A training manual for nursing assistants.* Glenview, IL: Association of Rehabilitation Nursing.

Vogelpohl, T., Beck, C., Heacock, P., & Mercer, S. (1996). I can do it dressing: Promoting independence through individualized strategies. *Journal of Gerontological Nursing, 22*(3), 39–42.

Walk, D., Fleishman, R., & Mendelson, J. (1999). Functional improvement of elderly residents of institutions. *Gerontologist, 39*(6), 720–728.

Waters, K. (1994). Getting dressed in the early morning: Styles of staff/patient interaction on rehabilitation hospital wards for elderly people. *Journal of Advanced Nursing, 19,* 239–247.

Winger, J., & Schirm, V. (1989). Managing aggressive elderly in long-term care. *Journal of Gerontological Nursing, 15*(2), 28–33.

Wolfe, S., Nordstrom, C., & Williams, K. (1998). The effect of enhancing self-efficacy prior to job training. *Journal of Social Behavior & Personality, 13*(4), 633–651.

CHAPTER 2

Staff Education and Motivation: Establishing the Restorative Care Philosophy

Barbara Resnick and Marjorie Simpson

Traditionally care of older adults has focused on providing care for these individuals, with an emphasis on safety and comfort during this stage of life. A restorative care philosophy changes that paradigm to focus not only on providing care for older adults, but on helping these individuals maximize and maintain their function. While nursing interventions are central to a successful restorative care program, it is essential that all persons working with an older adult follow the same philosophy. For example, a nursing assistant may diligently encourage an older individual all day to walk across the room to get his or her own water to drink, but in the evening, the housekeeper may cheerfully bring the individual a drink and even hold the cup and straw up to the individual's mouth. This undermines the restorative work that was previously done by the nursing assistant.

Establishing a restorative philosophy of care is best done by educating all caregivers and individuals who interact with older individuals about what restorative care is, what the benefits are for both older adults and caregivers, and what impact it can have on residents' quality of life (Table 2.1). Education should include opportunities for caregivers to ask questions and discuss their feelings about, for example, encouraging a 100-year-old woman to get up and walk to the dining room when she requests to lie in bed and be fed. In addition, there needs to be consensus between the caregivers and administration regarding work priorities. Rewards for work well done should be based on helping individuals participate in functional activities (i.e., the process) rather than on having all assigned patients bathed and dressed by a certain time (the outcome). Examples might include providing gift certificates monthly to

nursing assistants who walk the greatest number of patients to the dining room in a walk to dine program.

The adequacy of education and training systems will effect the implementation of a restorative philosophy of care. Carefully consider the education and training approaches you want to use, and evaluate what has been successful in the past. Caregivers may vary in what they know about restorative care and how they learn; therefore, different types of programs may be needed. Inservice programs or classroom education alone may not suffice. Walking rounds, in which education is incorporated into real care activities with older individuals may be a good way to reinforce information provided on restorative care. For example, teaching a nursing assistant specific restorative care techniques at an individual's bedside may be an effective learning technique.

When a nursing facility implements a restorative care philosophy, staff turnover is likely to be quite

TABLE 2.1 Overview of an Education Program for Restorative Care

1. Introduction to restorative care nursing with a strong focus on the new philosophy of care
2. Restorative care interventions: Transfers, ambulation and exercise, training activities, range of motion exercises, and splint/brace training
3. Restorative care interventions: Bathing, dressing, feeding, communication, and bowel/bladder training
4. Documentation of restorative care activities and review of interventions
5. Restorative care interventions: How to motivate the resident to participate in functional activities
6. Techniques to incorporate restorative care activities into regular daily care

high. Therefore, the facility should plan to orient new staff to the restorative care philosophy being implemented and ensure that they have the skills to provide this type of care. It may be useful to incorporate education about a restorative care philosophy into the orientation of all new staff in the facility. This training should focus on the general goals of restorative care— to maintain and optimize the function and quality of life of all residents. New staff should be informed that, unlike traditional care practice, care behaviors that focus on augmenting function will be reinforced in this facility. Mrs. B, for example, may not be fully bathed and dressed by 10:00 a.m. because she is being encouraged to perform much of these activities herself and it takes significantly longer to complete the task. The nursing assistant needs to know that he or she will be praised for facilitating this type of personal care, not reprimanded for not having Mrs. B bathed and dressed in time to go to the dining room for breakfast.

TRADITIONAL NURSING ASSISTANT TRAINING

In long-term care facilities the majority of the hands-on care is provided by nursing assistants, who receive only 75 hours of training in order to become certified (Feuerberg, 2001). Formal follow-up training is recommended; however, it is minimal and does not address the special care needs of older adults (Feuerberg, 2001). Consequently, nursing assistants are poorly prepared to meet the complex needs of older adults. In a large study of 440 nursing homes in Minnesota that examined the relationship between staffing levels of nursing personnel and older adult outcomes, Bliesmer and Smaylin (1998) found that licensed nursing hours were associated with less decline in function. This study suggests that the higher level of training that licensed nurses receive, versus the limited preparation of nursing assistants, prepares them to prevent functional decline in older adults. Therefore, continuing educational opportunities for nursing assistants that focus on aspects of care to promote independence will likely prevent some of the currently noted physical decline among older individuals.

NURSING ASSISTANT WORK-RELATED STRESS

Since 1985, the average number of activities of daily living (ADLs) with which an older adult in a long-term care setting required help to perform increased from 3.8 (out of 6) to 4.4. The average ratio of nursing assistants to older adults has not increased over time (Sahyoun, Pratt, Lentzner, Dey, & Robinson, 2001). Certain characteristics of the nursing assistant occupation result in high levels of job-related stress, turnover, and poor self-esteem (Kopiec, 2000). These include poor wages and benefits, poor recognition and appreciation (Parsons, Simmons, Penn, & Furlough, 2003), heavy workloads, a negative public image (National Citizens' Coalition for Nursing Home Reform, 2001), ongoing tensions between nurses and nursing assistants due to an intense division of labor (Rheaume, 2003; Schirm, Albanese, Garland, Gibson, & Blackmon, 2000), perceptions of being unappreciated and undervalued (Bowers, Esmond, & Jacobson, 2003), time pressure demands (Gonge, Jensen, & Bonde, 2002), and high psychological demands (Morgan, Semchuck, Stewart, & D'Arcy, 2002).

Working with older adults is physically strenuous and increases the risk of injuries to care providers. Musculoskeletal disorders are prevalent in nursing staff who have jobs with high physical demands (Josephson & Vingard, 1998; Trinkoff, Lipscomb, Geiger-Brown, Storr, & Brady, 2003), and time pressure demands (Gonge, Jensen, & Bonde, 2002; Lipscomb, Trinkoff, Geiger-Brown, & Brady, 2002). These musculoskeletal disorders have serious health implications for nursing assistants. Well-organized work, however, is associated with a decrease in time pressure demands and a decease in workload (Sinervo, 2000). Therefore, job-training interventions should include approaches aimed at improving organization and decreasing physical and psychological stress for nursing assistants.

SELF-EFFICACY AND JOB TRAINING

Very little research exists to support increased skills and knowledge for nursing assistants through job training (Almquist, Stein, Weiner, & Linn, 1981; Burgio, Allen-Burge et al. 2001; Cohn, Horgas, & Marsiske, 1990; Grabois & Coumbus, 1975). However, certain characteristics of job-training programs that promote learning and knowledge transfer. Training programs do consider individual characteristics such as self-efficacy, self-esteem, and motivation are more effective in enhancing job performance than those that do not consider these components of learning (Salas & Cannon-Bowers, 2001).

Using the self-efficacy framework is an effective way to enhance a job-training program or change job-related behavior. In a meta-analysis of training research, Colquitt, LePine, and Noe (2000) found that self-efficacy is a predictor of training motivation and training outcomes. Employees with high self-efficacy more effectively seek and utilize feedback obtained from managers and peers to improve their role clarity and job performance (Brown, Ganesan, & Challagalla, 2001). Additionally, employees with higher self-efficacy have lower job-related stress-strain and demonstrate more effective coping styles than employees with lower levels of self-efficacy (Jex, Bliese, Buzzell, & Primeau, 2001). Self-efficacy– based training interventions also reduce job performance anxiety (Martocchio, 1994), increase the beneficial effects of performance feedback (Karl, Olerykelly, & Martocchio, 1993), and reduce job turnover rates (Wolfe, Nordstrom, & Williams, 1998). Individuals with low baseline self-efficacy may actually have greater gains from job-training interventions than individuals with higher levels of self-efficacy (Gibson, 2001).

SELF-ESTEEM AND JOB PERFORMANCE

An individual's level of self-esteem has an impact on behavior and may play a role in coping with job-related stress. Self-esteem is defined as an individual's perception of his or her capabilities, successfulness, and worthiness (Ootim, 1998). In a longitudinal cohort study that measured self-esteem and perceived level of stress and coping in a group of 333 undergraduate nursing students, positive self-esteem was significantly related to proactive coping behaviors (p<.01). The professional socialization process in nursing is responsible for the development of professional self-esteem, and negative influence in the clinical setting can fragment an individual's professional self-esteem (Randle, 2001). In a study conducted by Kopiec (2000) that examined the work experiences of nursing assistants through focus group discussions and individual interviews with nursing assistants, the lack of professional support from nursing supervisory staff often depleted the self-esteem of nursing assistants. Although there is little research to support self-esteem as a factor in nursing assistants' job performance, interventions that increase professional self-esteem in nursing assistants may alter coping behaviors related to job stress.

The success of any intervention designed to improve nursing home care depends heavily on the receptiveness of the nurses and nursing assistants to learn new skills and on their motivation to use these skills regularly. Staff motivational systems such as behavioral supervision (Burgio & Burgio, 1990) have been used successfully, particularly to have nursing assistants implement interventions to improve quality of care. In one study (Stevens et al., 1998), behavioral supervision, in which nursing assistants are observed and provided with verbal feedback related to care activities, changed behavior of the nursing assistants and resulted in an increased amount of verbal interaction between nursing assistants and older adults.

TRAINING INTERVENTIONS TO INFLUENCE NURSING ASSISTANT BEHAVIOR

Several interventions have been developed to change behavior of nursing assistants and teach them to encourage the older adults they work with to increase their participation in ADLs. Beck and colleagues (Beck, Heacock, Rapp, & Mercer, 1993; Beck, Heacock, Mercer, Walls, Rapp, & Vogelpohl, 1995) tested Strategies to Promote Independence in Dressing (SPID), a training program that focuses on matching older adults' level of assistance needed with their underlying ability and provides some additional training on how nursing assistants can facilitate performance of ADLs. SPID also focused on the motivation of older adults and provided them with immediate reinforcers for successfully performing a dressing task (Vogelpohl et al., 1996). Blair (1996) developed and tested an intervention to encourage independence in functional activities using mutual goal setting and behavioral procedures (prompting, shaping, and providing reinforcement) to get older adults to engage in functional activities. Goal setting had a positive effect on older adults' self-care activities, and positive reinforcement was effective in motivating the older adults to perform self-care activities. Another intervention, "Self Care for Seniors" (Morris et al., 1999) incorporates five steps, including evaluating older adults' ability to perform self-care activities, establishing appropriate goals and a plan of care based on those abilities, and selecting environmental, communication, and motivational guidelines to assist the older adult in performance of self-care activities. Finally, an intervention that focused on training nursing assistants to increase communication between themselves and the older adults they work with had a positive effect on function, behavior, and social isolation of those older individuals (Allen-Burge, Stevens, & Burgio, 1999).

These studies all demonstrate that older adult–caregiver interactions that incorporate careful evaluation of the older adults' underlying ability, goal setting, and positive verbal encouragement can improve functional performance of older adults. None of the studies considered the outcome expectations of either the nursing assistants or the older adults with regard to restorative care activities. Unfortunately, in these and other studies (Remsburg, Palmer, Langford, & Mendelson, 1999; Schnelle, Cruise, Rahman & Ouslander, 1998) the nursing assistants exposed to the suggested interventions usually reverted back to preintervention behavior that continued to encourage dependency. Barriers to adhering to alternative care techniques included lack of motivation to continue the intervention, poor pay, minimal long-term benefits, insufficient training, insufficient recognition and support, inadequate staffing, workload, staff turnover, costs, and lack of perceived benefit (Beck, Ortigara, Mercer & Shue, 1999; Lekan-Rutledge, Palmer, & Belyea, 1998; Schnelle, Cruise et al., 1998). Strengthening the self-efficacy and outcome expectations of nursing assistants helps increase motivation and eliminates some of the barriers to implementing and maintaining a restorative care philosophy. The goal is to change beliefs and attitudes about restorative care and help nursing staff and nursing assistants to incorporate these activities into daily care.

USING A SELF-EFFICACY APPROACH

The theory of self-efficacy, as described in chapter 1, is the foundation of the Nursing Assistant Restorative Care Activities Intervention (NARCAI). This intervention focuses on helping to change beliefs, both self-efficacy and outcome expectations, related to restorative care activities. The informational sources suggested by Bandura (1997) are used to strengthen beliefs, as described in Table 2.2. The first step in implementing the NARCAI and this new philosophy of care, which focuses on function and maintaining function, is to identify a champion within the facility. The champion is essential to implementing the changes and keeping the staff focused and excited about the changes occurring. This champion may be the director of nursing, a staff nurse, a nursing assistant, an activi-

TABLE 2.2 Components of Nursing Assistant Restorative Care Activities

Source of Information	Techniques
Enactive mastery experience or successful performance of the activity of interest	Actual performance of restorative care activities during training and repeated continually as a way to increase confidence in capability
Verbal persuasion or verbal encouragement	Regular verbal encouragement and reinforcement for performance of restorative care activities
Vicarious experience	Role modeling or highlighting successful restorative care cases/ recognizing others for restorative care activities
Physiological and affective states	Decreasing the unpleasant sensations associated with restorative care activities such as anxiety about getting work completed, frustration with residents either for lack of motivation or slow response

ties staff member, or the administrator or medical director. With the help of the champion, the NARCAI can be used to implement and maintain a restorative care philosophy throughout the facility.

Self-efficacy is postulated by Bandura (1997) to be a major mediator of behavior and behavior change. Therefore, low self-efficacy expectations regarding a task or task domain will result in the avoidance of this kind of task (or situation). However, high self-efficacy expectations should increase the frequency of approach instead of avoidance behavior. Self-efficacy beliefs can be useful in understanding and predicting behavior or task performance. In addition, interventions designed to facilitate approach behavior are very effective because they increase individuals' expectations of self-efficacy with respect to the problematic, previously avoided, behavior. Furthermore, this concept has been widely applied and successfully used in educational and managerial settings. Self-efficacy expectations function particularly well as mediators between the assigned goal and actual performance, and boosted self-efficacy influences personal goals. Finally, both boosted self-efficacy and personal goals have an influence on performance (Resnick & Simpson, 2003).

THE BENEFIT OF SELF-EFFICACY

Prior research (Bandura, 1995) supports the important benefit of self-efficacy with regard to how people feel (affect), think (cognition), and act (motivation and behavior). In terms of affect, a low sense of self-efficacy is associated with depression, anxiety, and helplessness. Individuals with low self-efficacy also have low self-esteem and harbor pessimistic thoughts about their accomplishments and personal development. In terms of cognition, a strong sense of competence facilitates cognitive processes in a variety of settings, including quality of decision making and academic achievement. In terms of preparing action, self-related cognitions are a major ingredient of the motivation process. Self-efficacy levels can enhance or impede motivation. People with high self-efficacy choose to perform more challenging tasks (Bandura, 1995). They set themselves higher goals and stick to them. Actions are preshaped in thought, and people anticipate either optimistic or pessimistic scenarios in line with their level of self-efficacy. Once an action has been taken, people with high self-efficacy invest more effort and persist longer than those who are low in self-efficacy. When setbacks occur, they recover more quickly and maintain the commitment to their goals. Self-efficacy also allows people to select challenging settings, explore their environments, and create new environments.

A strong sense of efficacy is needed to remain task oriented in the face of pressing situational demands, failures, and setbacks that have significant repercussions. Indeed, when people are faced with the tasks of managing difficult environmental demands under taxing circumstances, those who are beset by self-doubts about their efficacy become more and more erratic in their analytic thinking, they lower their aspirations, and the quality of their performance deteriorates. In contrast, those who maintain a resilient sense of efficacy set themselves challenging goals and use good analytic thinking, which pays off in performance accomplishments.

EDUCATION OF CAREGIVERS

Will education alone change behavior? It's not likely. However, it is important to educate staff about restorative care, with a particular focus on the benefits of these activities so that outcome expectations for restorative care are strengthened. The focus of this education is not simply to provide information but really to change beliefs. To help nurses, nursing assistants, and administrative, medical, activities, and housekeeping staff to understand and believe in the important benefits associated with maintenance of function in older adults. Consider the scenario of Mrs. Jones going to the dining room. Mrs. Jones is capable of walking the short distance but likes to go in a wheelchair. The nursing assistant, being a fantastic proponent of restorative care, has set Mrs. Jones up to walk down the hallway to the dining room. Mrs. Jones is somewhat disgruntled about it but is grudgingly adhering. Maggie from housekeeping happens by and sees Mrs. Jones struggling a bit and offers to have her sit in the wheelchair and be pushed. Maggie has just undermined the entire restorative care attempt with Mrs. Jones. Clearly, the importance of team education regarding the philosophy and benefit of restorative care is essential.

The educational component of the NARCAI includes a series of six weekly 30-minute interactive self-efficacy based training sessions that focus on the philosophy of restorative care and motivating older adults to participate in restorative care activities. Specifically, the NARCAI training programs focus on the philosophy of care that drives a restorative care nursing program and the specific benefits of restorative care for older adults and staff, techniques to motivate and strengthen self-efficacy, outcome expectations for older adults to perform restorative care activities, and the specific skills and techniques needed to perform restorative care activities (Fleishell & Resnick, 1999; Resnick & Fleishell, 1999). Training can easily be provided in each facility by the identified champion of restorative care, the director of nursing or of nursing education, or the geriatric nurse practitioner. The weekly recommended inservices, to be used as a kickoff to implementing a restorative care philosophy, are outlined in Table 2.3, further detailed in Figure 2.1 (Power Point presentations), and briefly described below.

TABLE 2.3   List of Weekly Classes for 6-Week Training Program

Week 1:	Introduction to Restorative Care Nursing: focus on the new philosophy of care
Week 2:	Restorative Care Activities: Transfers, ambulation and exercise training activities, range of motion exercises, and splint/brace training
Week 3:	Restorative Care Interventions: Bathing, dressing, feeding, communication, and bowel/bladder training.
Week 4:	Documentation
Week 5:	Motivation: How to motivate the resident to participate in functional activities
Week 6:	Incorporating Restorative Care Activities Into Regular Daily Care

Week 1:

Introduction to Restorative Care

What is restorative care?

Restorative nursing care focuses on the restoration and/or maintenance of physical function and helps older adults to perform their own personal activities such as bathing, dressing, and walking and other daily exercise and encourages them to do as much as

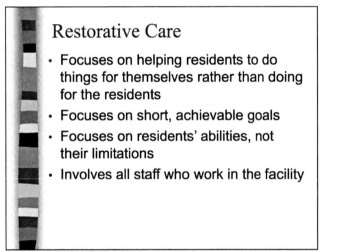

Restorative Care

- Focuses on helping residents to do things for themselves rather than doing for the residents
- Focuses on short, achievable goals
- Focuses on residents' abilities, not their limitations
- Involves all staff who work in the facility

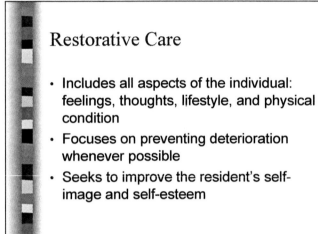

Restorative Care

- Includes all aspects of the individual: feelings, thoughts, lifestyle, and physical condition
- Focuses on preventing deterioration whenever possible
- Seeks to improve the resident's self-image and self-esteem

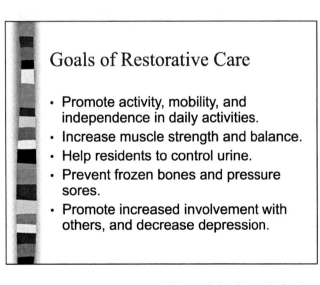

Goals of Restorative Care

- Promote activity, mobility, and independence in daily activities.
- Increase muscle strength and balance.
- Help residents to control urine.
- Prevent frozen bones and pressure sores.
- Promote increased involvement with others, and decrease depression.

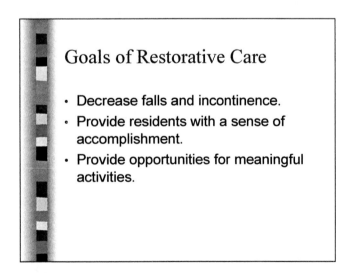

Goals of Restorative Care

- Decrease falls and incontinence.
- Provide residents with a sense of accomplishment.
- Provide opportunities for meaningful activities.

Figure 2.1 PowerPoint Presentations for Inservice Education.

Benefits of Restorative Care

- Psychological:
  - better mood
  - better overall quality of life
  - feel like they have accomplished something
- Physical
  - perform daily activities better
  - stronger
  - good for the heart and cardiovascular system

Specific Restorative Care Activities Include:

Encouraging and getting a resident to:

- Participate in his/her own bathing and dressing
- Walk to the dining room
- Lift weights while watching TV

Restorative Care Activities

- Moving all extremities to help the resident keep joints moving
- Eating independently/or as independently as possible
- Wearing a splint or support that helps the resident to keep his or her extremities in the right position and also to do as much as possible independently (large-grip eating utencils)

Examples of Restorative Care

Mrs. Jones has had a stroke and so her balance is not perfect. She is able to get up out of the wheelchair alone and to walk with a walker as long as someone is by her side.

- What restorative care activities might you do with her?
- How could you implement this into daily activities?

Examples of Restorative Care

Mrs. Green has very bad arthritis so it is hard for her to hold a fork or spoon.

- What restorative care activities might you do with her?
- How could you implement this into daily activities?

Figure 2.1 (*continued*)

Week 2: Restorative Care Activities

Bed mobility, positioning, transfer, and ambulation

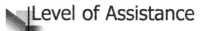

Level of Assistance

- Independent: Patient able to perform without the assistance of another individual or without adaptive equipment
- Independent with adaptive equipment
- Setup: Independent after setup of adaptive equipment
- Supervision or standby assistance: Requires staff presence during activity for safety
- Cueing: Step-by-step instructions for activity Provided by staff

Level of Assistance continued

- Minimum assistance: Resident performs 75% or more of activity. Needs only incidental help such as contact guard or steadying.
- Moderate assistance: Resident performs 50%–74% of activity. Hands-on assistance required.
- Maximum assistance: Resident performs 25%–49% of the activity. Weight bearing assistance is required.

-

Good Alignment and Positioning Basic Principles

- Purpose: Ensure that the joints are in their functional position and not abnormally flexed or extended.
- Equipment: Use rolled towels, small sandbags, pillows, or specific positioning devices for the bed or chair.

Elements of a Therapeutic Position

- The spine is straight.
- The head and neck are straight (can be supported by a pillow).
- Arms are at side in neutral position with elbows extended and palms down.
- Feet are at right angles to the legs to prevent foot-drop (a footboard can be used).
- Fingers are kept straight by placing a rolled washcloth, finger or hand positioning device, or splint in the hands.

Supine Position

- On back, a small flat pillow supports the head, neck, and upper shoulders.
- The arms are in a neutral position at the side with elbows extended and palms down, or abducted with pad elevating the forearm and hand.
- Legs are straight with a pillow under the calves to relieve pressure from heels.

Figure 2.1 (*continued*)

Prone Position

- On the abdomen, head is turned to one side with a small pillow under the head and another between the chest and the umbilicus to relieve pressure on the chest and breasts.
- Hips and knees are extended and supported by pillows.
- Feet and toes are supported by another pillow, arms flexed over head or extended along the body in a neutral position.

 ## Lateral Position

- Position on side with head straight with spine.
- Place pillow or wedge against the back.
- Place pillow under the head, neck, and upper shoulder.
- Place pillow under top arm and top leg.
- Flex the bottom arm; use footboard or foot splints to prevent foot-drop.

 ## Sitting Position

- Keep body positioned in straight alignment.
- Support the head and neck with pillows if needed to prevent hyperextension or flexion.
- Use armrests or pillow to support arms and hands, place feet on floor or use footrests to prevent foot-drop and edema.
- Ensure that knees extend past the edge of

 ## Commonly Occurring Deformities/Contractures

- External rotation of the hip: The hip rotates outward when the patient is in a supine position.
- Fixed plantar flexion (foot-drop): The feet drop downward.
- Joints such as shoulders, knees, and hips become stiff and do not extend

 ## Other Equipment

- Trochanter rolls: A bath blanket or flannel sheet is folded lengthwise into thirds and positioned beneath the resident's hips from the top of the iliac crest to approximately 6 inches above the knee to prevent outward rotation of the hip when the resident is in a supine position.

 ## Other Equipment continued

- Hand rolls: A rolled washcloth or soft rubber ball is placed in the hand to keep the hand in a slightly flexed position.
- Foot supports: Used as an alternative to a footboard. Can be a blanket-covered box, resting leg splints, or high-top sneakers. Be sure to check for pressure areas and exercise the feet to maintain muscle tone, strength, and joint range.

Figure 2.1 (*continued*)

Restorative Care

- Prevents further impairment and maintains present function
- Builds muscle strength
- Maintains joint function and prevents deformity
- Stimulates circulation
- Builds tolerance and endurance

Types of Exercises to Maintain Function

- Passive: Exercise that is done without the assistance of the patient.
- Active Assistance: Carried out by the patient with help to encourage normal muscle function. The distal part of the joint should be supported while the patient is encouraged to take the joint actively through its range of motion.

Types of Exercises continued

- Active: Exercise that is done by the patient without any assistance to increase muscle strength. The joint is moved through a full range of motion without assistance. Includes turning in bed, pushing up in bed, or transferring.
- Resistive: Active exercise carried out by the patient working against resistance produced by another individual or mechanical means to increase muscle strength and improve functioning.

Range of Motion

- Passive range of motion should be performed on all chairbound and bedbound residents.
- Residents are better able to move joints immediately following passive range of motion. Therefore, it is best to perform range of motion prior to a.m. and p.m. care.
- Range of motion will decrease a resident's risk of injuries and bone fractures because it improves joint function and overall mobility.

Instructions for Range of Motion (ROM)

- Perform while the resident is lying in bed.
- Applying ice or a warm moist towel for 20 minutes, or topical analgesics such as Bengay prior to ROM will help decrease discomfort.
- Slowly move each joint until you feel resistance.
- Range each joint three times.
- ROM takes less than 5 minutes, significantly improves joint functioning, and makes providing care easier.

Range of Motion of Joints

- Adduction
- Abduction
- Opposition
- Extension
- Flexion
- Elevation (shrugging shoulders)

Figure 2.1 (*continued*)

Splints and Braces

- Purpose: Properly position joints and maintain joint function, reduce spacticity, prevent contractures.
- NA responsibility:
  - Apply and remove splint according to schedule (usually 2 hours on, 2 hours off).
  - Assess the splint area for pressure spots or irritation. Reddened areas should resolve within 15 minutes of removing the splint.
  - Keep the splint and the limb clean (wash splint with warm, not hot, soapy water).
  - Document the splint-wearing time.

 Prosthesis

- Artificial legs, feet, or hands are attached to limbs that have had amputations.
- Provide support during ambulation.
- NA responsibilities:
  - Check the device for any broken or missing parts or problems.
  - Assist the resident to apply and remove the prosthesis.

 Ambulation/Mobility

- Walking alone or with the use of walker, cane, or staff assistance; or wheeling in a wheelchair

 Gait Belts

- Promote ambulation and mobility by providing increased security for resident and staff.
- Reduce the risk of injury to residents and staff from holding onto resident's limbs and skin.
- Place the belt over clothing and around the waist to fit snugly (the NA should be able to place two fingers inside the belt).

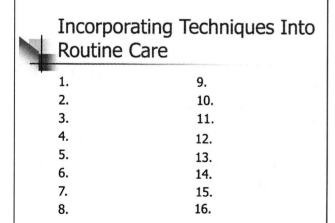

Incorporating Techniques Into Routine Care

1.
2.
3.
4.
5.
6.
7.
8.

9.
10.
11.
12.
13.
14.
15.
16.

Figure 2.1 (*continued*)

Week 3: Restorative Care Interventions

Bathing, dressing, feeding, communication, and bowel and bladder training

Methods to Ensure Restorative Care Success

- Know the specific interventions/goals for the resident.
- Don't expect consistent performance each day. Work with the resident the same time each day.
- Include family members as much as possible.
- Remove distractions from the environment (turn off TV).

Restorative Care Activities

- Follow the short-term goals and NA approaches posted in the resident's room.
- Have the resident do as much as possible for him- or herself.
- Cue the resident and provide step-by-step instructions.
- Break tasks down into smaller steps so that the resident can complete care him- or herself.
- Encourage and motivate the resident throughout care.

Bathing Adaptive Equipment

- Shower chair
- Handheld shower head
- Washing mitts and extension sponges
- Soap on a rope or liquid soap

Dressing

- Wear personal clothing that signifies an active lifestyle.
- Clothing should be clean and attractive to promote the resident's positive self-image.
- Choose clothing that is easy to apply: loose necklines and sleeves, large buttons or Velcro, front-opening, loose undergarments, elastic waistbands, bras with front closure. Consider clothing one size larger.

Dressing Adaptive Equipment

- Long and lead shoe horns
- Sock pullers
- Velcro closures
- Button hooks
- Zipper pulls

Figure 2.1 (*continued*)

Dressing Techniques

- Allow the resident to choose his or her own clothing.
- Consider sitting and standing balance. Develop methods for dressing in bed or chair if balance is inadequate.
- Develop an appropriate dressing sequence and practice it with the resident.

Restorative Grooming

- Includes personal hygiene (application of deodorant, lotion, or powder), oral hygiene, hair care, shaving, applying makeup, applying glasses or hearing aids.
- Make sure the resident is positioned well with equipment and assistive devices in reach.
- Follow the same routine every day.

Grooming Equipment

- Electric toothbrush or water-pic
- Electric razors, especially if taking anticoagulant medication
- Suction cups to stabilize cosmetic jars to counter tops
- Handheld or countertop mirrors

Restorative Feeding

- Purpose is to increase independence.
- Use assistive devices such as weighted utensils.
- Serve food that requires little cutting.
- Provide hand-over-hand assistance instead of spoon feeding.
- Provide larger portions if spilling food is a problem.

Restorative Feeding continued

- Set up food and utensils and cut food into small pieces.
- Season the food the way the resident likes it.
- Fill the spoon half full.
- Alternate between liquids and solid foods.
- Use small bites of food.
- Allow the resident time to eat.

Feeding Equipment

- Longer straws when ROM is limited
- Cups with lids
- Wrist weights to reduce tremors
- Structured food placement for the blind
- Plates with high sides to make it easier to scoop food

Figure 2.1 (*continued*)

Restorative Eating and Swallowing

- Purpose: facilitate chewing and swallowing.
- Sit next to the resident and use hand‾over‾ hand assistance.
- Present food horizontally below the mouth, place the spoon on the midportion of the tongue, and press down lightly.
- Gently stroke the throat or press on the root of the tongue to increase swallowing.
- Provide mouth care before and after meals to increase salivation and prevent aspiration of food particles.

Signs of Dysphagia

- Coughing or choking during or after meals
- Long time to eat meals
- Hoarseness or gurgly voice during or after meal
- Pain when swallowing
- Heartburn or indigestion
- Food coming out through the nose
- Excessive drooling
- Frequent respiratory infections
- Weight loss

Communication Training

- Establish a means of communicating with the resident if at all possible (speech, eye blinks, head nods, finger or eye movements, communication board, yes/no answers).
- Face resident and make direct eye contact.
- Speak slowly and distinctly with normal tone.
- Use appropriate gestures.
- Allow the resident time to process the information.
- Ask for clarification if needed.
- Try to find meaning in jargon or nonsense language.

Communication Training for Cognitive Impairment

- Proceed from simple to complex, promoting success along the way. Repeat commands.
- Be patient and consistent with memory training and allow for extra response time.
- Plan activities during the resident's peak periods of alertness.
- Divide tasks into short 15-minute segments and do not overstimulate.
- Use sensory stimulation (vision, hearing, smell, taste, or touch).
- Converse with resident while providing care.

Compensating for Hearing and Visual Changes

- Provide visual cues.
- Use simple lettering with high-contrast black against white.
- Avoid the use of greens, blues, and purples due to the yellowing effect of the lens.
- Avoid glare (use matte finish instead of glossy finish).

Toileting

- Independence relies on several cognitive and physical processes:
  - Ability to recognize the signal to eliminate
  - Remembering the actions to take when the signal is sensed
  - Physical function, which can make it difficult for the resident to get to the toilet "in time"

Figure 2.1 (*continued*)

Causes of Urinary Incontinence

- D—Delirium or confusional state
- I—Infection, UTI
- A—Atropic urethritis/vaginitis
- P—Pharmaceuticals
- P—Psychologic, especially depression
- E—Endocrine (hypercalcemia, hyperglycemia)
- R—Restricted mobility
- S—Stool impaction/constipation

Bladder Training

- Follow voiding schedule. Place resident on the toilet at specified times.
- Avoid caffeine and alcohol.
- Encourage fluids throughout the day. Restricting fluids can cause dehydration.
- Provide verbal cues and encouragement.

Factors That Affect Normal Bowel Function

- Diet: High fiber with good fluid intake essential.
- Exercise: Impaired mobility and function may prevent a resident's ability to toilet.
- Time, positioning, and place: When the urge to defecate is felt, people must respond in a timely manner.

Incorporating Techniques Into Routine Care

1.	9.
2.	10.
3.	11.
4.	12.
5.	13.
6.	14.
7.	15.
8.	16.

Figure 2.1 (*continued*)

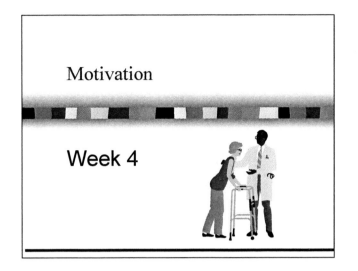

Motivation

Week 4

What is Motivation?

- Motivation comes from within the individual and refers to the need, drive, or desire to act in a certain way to achieve a certain end.
- Motivation is behavior specific, and must be considered for any activity.

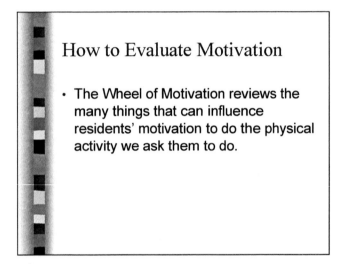

How to Evaluate Motivation

- The Wheel of Motivation reviews the many things that can influence residents' motivation to do the physical activity we ask them to do.

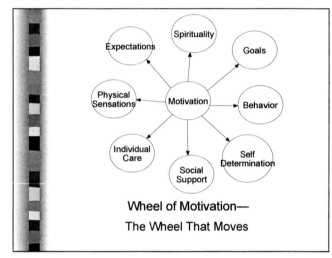

Wheel of Motivation—

The Wheel That Moves

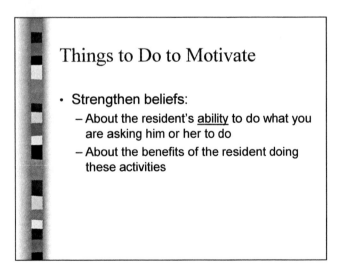

Things to Do to Motivate

- Strengthen beliefs:
  - About the resident's <u>ability</u> to do what you are asking him or her to do
  - About the benefits of the resident doing these activities

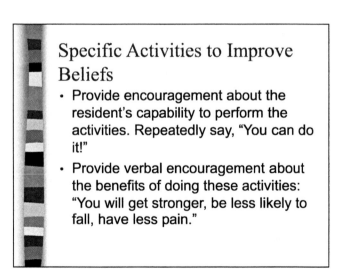

Specific Activities to Improve Beliefs

- Provide encouragement about the resident's capability to perform the activities. Repeatedly say, "You can do it!"
- Provide verbal encouragement about the benefits of doing these activities: "You will get stronger, be less likely to fall, have less pain."

Figure 2.1 (*continued*)

Specific Activities to Improve Beliefs

- Give the resident examples of role models (other residents who successfully perform the activity).
- Encourage actual performance/practice doing the activity—bathing, walking.
- REVIEW, REVIEW, REVIEW the benefits.

Restoring Health and Function

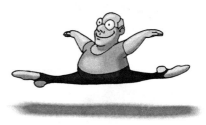

Restorative Care

- **Focuses on preventing disability and helping older adults to improve and maintain their physical and psychological health so that they can continue to function as independently as possible**

What Can Restorative Care Do?

- **Improve strength and maximum aerobic capacity**
- **Prevent disease**
- **Decrease risk of falling**
- **Reduce physical disability**
- **Improve sleep**
- **Enhance mood and well-being**

Restorative Care May

Help you become physically fit by improving your

- **muscle strength (force the muscles to exert)**
- **muscle endurance (the ability of the muscle to keep repeating an activity without getting tired)**

Restorative Care May:

Help you become physically fit by improving your

- **flexibility (the ability to move your joints—arms, legs, neck, and back)**
- **balance (the ability to maintain your body in a standing position)**

Figure 2.1 (*continued*)

Participating in Personal Care Activities Can:

- Strengthen your muscles and bones
- Improve your flexibility
- Improve your overall feeling of well-being

Restoring Function Is Helped By:

- Increasing overall activity
- Moving, moving, and moving!

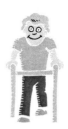
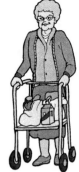

A Balanced Activity Program Includes:

- Aerobic exercises—walking
- Resistive exercises—weight training with some type of hand weights
- Flexibility training—muscle stretching

INCREASE YOUR ACTIVITY BY:

- Decreasing time spent in a wheelchair
- Walking to the bathroom or dining room
- Doing as much of your own personal care as possible

Incorporate Exercise Into Your Daily Activity

- Moving yourself around in bed
- Getting up and down from the bed or chair frequently (every half hour)
- Walking instead of using the wheelchair
- Participating in daily activities

HOW TO KEEP WITH IT!

- Set up a regular time to exercise
- And get yourself to stick to that schedule

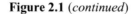

Figure 2.1 (*continued*)

**RESTORATIVE CARE
SHOULD BE:**

· **Realistic—don't set goals
that you can't meet!**

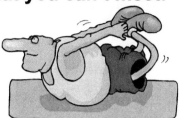

**RESTORATIVE ACTIVITIES
SHOULD BE**

· ENJOYABLE....
  – WALK WITH A FRIEND.
  – WALK TO A FRIEND.
  – LAUGH AND SMILE.
  – MAKE IT FUN!

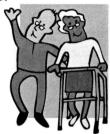

**OVERCOME THE CHALLENGES
TO PERFORMING RESTORATIVE
ACTIVITIES**

· "THERE IS NO PLACE TO DO
  THESE ACTIVITIES"
  – YOU CAN DO THESE ACTIVITIES
    RIGHT HERE.
  – SET DAILY SCHEDULE AND STICK TO
    IT!

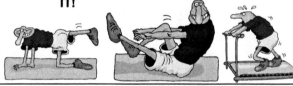

**OVERCOME THE CHALLENGES
TO PERFORMING RESTORATIVE
ACTIVITIES**

· "I AM TOO OLD TO
  EXERCISE OR TO DO
  PERSONAL CARE
  ACTIVITIES."

**OVERCOME THE CHALLENGES
TO PERFORMING RESTORATIVE
ACTIVITIES**

· "I'm not given enough time."
  –Relax and know there is no
   rush to get these activities
   done!

**OVERCOME THE CHALLENGES
TO PERFORMING RESTORATIVE
ACTIVITIES**

· "I FEEL TOO TIRED TO
  EXERCISE OR PERFORM
  PERSONAL CARE."

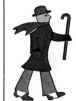
  –The activity will give you energy.
   Try it and see!

Figure 2.1 (*continued*)

OVERCOME THE CHALLENGES TO PERFORMING RESTORATIVE ACTIVITIES

- **"I have too much pain to exercise or perform personal care activities."**
  - Pain medication and other treatments can help control pain to get you started. And exercise can help prevent future pain.

OVERCOME THE CHALLENGES TO PERFORMING RESTORATIVE ACTIVITIES

- **"I don't know what to do."**
  - We will teach you the exact activities and exercises that will help you.

OVERCOME THE CHALLENGES TO PERFORMING RESTORATIVE ACTIVITIES

- **"I'm worried about getting hurt."**
  - The exercises and activity given to you are ones that you can do safely. Exercise will strengthen your bones and muscles and is the best way to prevent a fall.

OVERCOME THE CHALLENGES TO PERFORMING RESTORATIVE ACTIVITIES

- **I can't remember what to do."**
  - The recommended activities or exercises are written down for you. Just use your calendar and goal sheet.

Decrease the Unpleasant Physical Sensations (pain, fear)

- Make sure the resident gets pain medications to relieve discomfort.
- Use alternative ways to get rid of pain such as heat/ice.
- Have resident talk about his or her pain or fear associated with the activity—assume he or she has some unpleasant feelings during activity.

Decrease the Unpleasant Sensations

- Help the resident develop a more realistic attitude to the pain—i.e., pain will not hurt them/pain doesn't mean they shouldn't move.
- Use relaxation and distraction techniques.
- Help the resident overcome fear by actually performing the activity.

Figure 2.1 (*continued*)

Individualized Care

- Help the residents know you REALLY care about them!

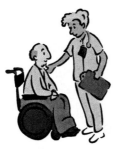

Individualized Care

- Be kind and caring to the resident—despite all things, smile and be nice.
- Use humor.
- GET EXCITED with the resident when he or she does any of the activities you recommend (bathe, dress, walk to the dining room).

Individualized Care

- Give positive feedback (a hug, a kiss) after the resident performs a desired activity (walks to the bathroom or dining room).
- Recognize individual needs and differences by, for example, setting a rest period, or providing a favorite snack.

Spirituality

- Encourage the resident to participate in traditional religious activities as desired.
- Spend time with the resident just listening, in particular, have him or her talk about life experiences.
- Encourage spiritual experiences: pets, children, friends, prayer.

Social Support—Help From Others

- Encourage involvement with others—family and friends, other residents, and staff.
- Encourage family and other visitors to verbally encourage/reinforce the resident for bathing, dressing, or walking to the dining room (or whatever the restorative goals are).
- Include visits with family/friends as a goal.

Basic Personality

- Recognize that some residents are just determined and motivated and will do all of the activities you recommend!

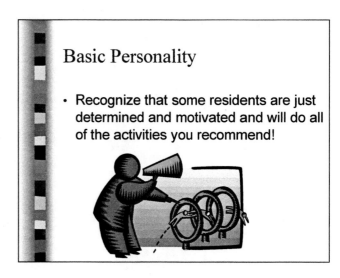

Figure 2.1 (*continued*)

Goal Identification

- Develop appropriate realistic goals with the resident.
- Set goals that can be met in a short time frame—daily or weekly.
- Set goals that are challenging but that the resident can REALLY achieve in a reasonable time frame.

Figure 2.1 (*continued*)

Week 5:
Documentation

Documentation: WHY?

- Generally, the recommendation (from the federal government) is for restorative care to be performed for 15 minutes at least 6 out of 7 days per week.
- BUT, we don't really know if 15 minutes is enough time for the resident to have a benefit or not.
- SO, to learn about the benefits of restorative care and how much time we spend providing restorative care, it is important for us to document care.

Goals and Approaches

- Long-term goals: The highest level of functioning that the resident can achieve over a long period of time with restorative care.
- Short-term goals: Goals that the resident is currently working toward. Short-term goals should progressively lead to meeting the long-term goal.
- Nursing assistant approaches: Approaches that NAs will use to help residents meet their short-term goals.

Example of Goals and Approaches

- Long-term goal: Walk independently with a rolling walker.
- Short-term goals: Walk to the dining room twice a day for meals.
- NA approaches:
  - Use a rolling walker.
  - Use a one-person minimal assistance.
  - Allow the resident to sit in a chair and rest half way for several minutes.

Long-Term and Short-Term Goals

- Long-term goal: Walk independently with a rolling walker.
- Short-term goals:
  - Walk ½ way to dining room twice a day.
  - Walk all the way to dining room twice a day.
  - Walk to dining room and back twice a day.
  - Walk to all activities and to the dining room for all meals.

Modifying Short-Term Goals and NA Approaches

- Nursing assistants may alter NA approaches to help residents meet short-term goals. If you come up with a creative way of helping a resident, use it!
- Nursing assistants may alter short-term goals and make them more challenging for residents when they have met the short-term goal or when the short-term goal activity becomes too easy.

Figure 2.1 (*continued*)

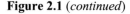

Example of Altering Goals

Established ST goal:
- Resident will walk ½ way to the dining room twice a day.

Approaches:
- Use one -person Assist.
- Use a rolling walker.

NA altered goal:
- The NA discovers that the resident can walk all of the way to the dining room for meals if he/she sits and rests half way for a few minutes.

Documentation

- A monthly calendar will be provided for you in the resident's room. One calendar will be for the daytime nursing assistant and one will be for the evening nursing assistant.
- The restorative care activity to be done will be written on the goal form.

Documentation

- So, if you walk the resident to the dining room every day at lunch and it takes 10 minutes each way, you would write 20 minutes.
- If you work with a resident in the morning to wash his/her upper body and put on a shirt (that is the goal) and it takes 15 minutes.

Documentation

- You will also be asked to fill out on the calendar the reason why you can't or didn't do the restorative care activity:
  - The resident may refuse.
  - You may forget.
  - You may feel you didn't have the time.
  - The resident may have to go out.

Calendar Documentation

- Circle the number of minutes spent performing restorative care.
- Fill in your initials.
- Write in the restorative care activity or the reason why restorative care wasn't performed.

Sun	Mon	Tues	Wed	Thur	Fri	Sat
Minutes: 5 20 10 30 15 40 Other min __ Initials: MS Activity: walked to dining room	Minutes: 5 20 10 30 15 40 Other min __ Initials ___ Activity:	Minutes: 5 20 10 30 15 40 Other min __ Initials ___ Activity:	Minutes: 5 20 10 30 15 40 Other min __ Initials ___ Activity:	Minutes: 5 20 10 30 15 40 Other min __ Initials ___ Activity:	Minutes: 5 20 10 30 15 40 Other min __ Initials ___ Activity:	Minutes: 5 20 10 30 15 40 Other min __ Initials ___ Activity:

Restorative Care Flowsheet

- A restorative care flowsheet will be kept in a binder at the nurses station.
- Write in the number of minutes spent performing restorative care for each activity of daily living.
- Sign your initials.

Figure 2.1 (*continued*)

Review of Restorative Care Activities

- All residents will have goals set by the restorative care nurse.
- Goals will be written on the goal form and placed in the resident's room.
- Goals will include both short- and long-term goals.
- Day shift and evening shift calendars will be placed in the resident's room to record what restorative care activities have been done.
- Sign off the restorative care flowsheet.

When to Notify the Restorative Care Nurse

- When long-term goals or short-term goals are met so that new goals can be developed.
- When you have altered short-term goals or NA approaches to make restorative care more challenging for the resident.
- When the resident is unable to perform the short-term goal activity.

Key Points

- Promote independence and functional performance by incorporating restorative care activities into all routine care for all of the residents.
- Focus on long-term goals, short-term goals, and nursing assistant approaches when these forms are posted in a resident's room.
- Use the goal forms, the calendar, and the restorative care poster to help motivate residents to participate in their care.

Figure 2.1 (*continued*)

Week 6: Incorporating Restorative Care Activities Into Regular Daily Care

Different Approaches to Care: Do "With" the Resident Instead of "For" the Resident

The "task" approach

- Staff focus on completing tasks as the most important part of care.
- Staff complete tasks for the resident with little or no involvement of the resident.
- No opportunity for improvement in functioning for the resident.
- No growth or learning opportunities for the resident or family members.

The "person" approach

- Enables the resident to do for him- herself as much as possible.
- Care benefits the resident.
- Staff provide physical and verbal cues to help the residents.
- Staff provide setup of adaptive equipment.
- Staff use hand-over-hand assistance during care.

Doing What Is Best for the Resident

- Restorative care:
  - Promotes functional performance and prevents disability.
  - Improves and maintains physical and psychological health.
  - Allows older adults to function as independently as possible.
  - Promotes dignity and well-being.

Benefits of Restorative Care to Nursing Assistants

- Restorative care enables nursing assistants to advance their skills and provide care that is therapeutic and more meaningful.
- As residents improve their functioning, there is less physical demand on the staff and less risk of on-the-job injuries.
- Restorative care is just as important as the medications and other treatments that the residents receive. You make a difference with the care you provide!

Incorporating Restorative Care into Bed Mobility and Transfers

- Allow residents to turn themselves over in bed and pull themselves up in bed using the bedrails as an assistive device. Assist only as needed.
- Remind residents to turn and reposition themselves every two hours.
- Keep the bed in the lowest possible position to make transfers easier for the resident.
- Remind and assist residents to use their walkers to transfer in and out of bed.
- Give the resident time and support during transfers. Many older adults become lightheaded or dizzy if they change positions too quickly.

Ambulation

- Make sure the resident is wearing proper footwear that offers support and prevents slipping.
- Incorporate ambulation into routine activities.
  - Walk residents to the bathroom and shower/tub room.
  - Walk residents to the dining room and to the activity room.
  - Have residents push other residents who are wheelchair bound and unable to wheel themselves.

Figure 2.1 (*continued*)

Incorporating Restorative Care Into Bathing, Dressing, and Grooming

- Set up one resident and let him or her begin bathing while you go to set up another resident.
- Provide rest periods if needed (bathing before breakfast and dressing after breakfast).
- Provide supervision and cueing to resident while you make the bed, change linens, put away bathing equipment.

Incorporating Restorative Care Into Mealtime

- Cut food up into pieces that are easier to manage.
- Place a piece of food or a cup into the resident's hand.
- Keep the tray in front of the resident even if he or she claims to be finished. Older adults will "pick" at food or accept more food after they have rested for a few minutes.
- Remove TV or radio noise from the room. Residents can easily become overstimulated and refuse to eat in an environment that is not calm.
- Sit next to the resident and talk to him or her during mealtime.

Incorporating Communication and Cognitive Training Into Routine Care

- Talk to residents during all care encounters.
- Ask them questions about family members, pictures in their room, or special events in their life.
- Use simple words and phrases.
- Be patient and give them time to respond to your questions.

Incorporating Bowel and Bladder Training Into Routine Care

- Toilet residents when you are walking them to and from the dining room or activities room. Remember that eating a meal often stimulates the urge to urinate or move bowels.
- Toilet residents before starting a.m. or p.m. care.
- Many older adults may need to urinate in the early morning between 4 a.m. and 6 a.m. A resident who is trying to climb out of bed at this time may be trying to get to the bathroom.
- Don't forget to encourage fluids.

Top 10 Reasons to Incorporate Restorative Care Into Routine Care Activities

- It is a great way to establish a routine for the residents.
- Combining tasks makes your job easier.
- Restorative care will improve residents' functioning.
- Higher functioning residents require less strenuous care.
- You have less risk of injuring yourself from lifting and pulling residents.

Top 10 continued

- You have less chance of injuring residents from lifting and pulling.
- Residents have fewer falls and skin tears.
- Family members feel more confident about the care that you provide.
- Residents feel better about themselves.

Figure 2.1 (*continued*)

#1 Reason to Provide Restorative Care

Restorative care is the highest quality of care that you can provide. It makes residents healthier both physically and mentally. You are making a difference by doing what is best for the residents.

Case Study #1

- Mrs. S is a resident who has been working very hard with PT and OT after being hospitalized for a hip fracture. She has just been discharged from PT and is able to ambulate with a walker and standby assistance for 50 feet.
- Just before lunch, you tell her that you will help her walk to the dining room. She tells you that she is feeling tired and would like to get back into bed to eat her lunch.
- The restorative care schedule indicates that Mrs. S is to ambulate with her walker and standby assistance to the dining room twice a day.

Case Study #2

- Mrs. Z has been in your facility for a long time. She used to do a lot for herself, but lately she has been more confused and does not seem able to perform even the simplest task.
- The restorative care nurse has written up a treatment plan for her that includes cueing her and offering some assistance while she is bathing and dressing.
- You have set Mrs. Z up in the shower with every thing that she needs to wash herself, but she just sits there looking like she is unable to do anything for herself.

Case Study #3

- You have been providing restorative ambulation for Mrs. M for 5 weeks. She usually tells you that she doesn't want to walk with her walker and would prefer for you to wheel her in her wheelchair to the dining room. You have always been very successful in motivating Mrs. M to ambulate by telling her, "You can do it," and telling her jokes and stories to make her laugh. In the end she has always walked to the dining room despite her initial protest.

Case Study #3 continued

- You go into Ms. M's room to help her walk to the dining room for lunch as you do each day. When you enter her room, her nephew is visiting with her. Ms. M says to him, "Here she is again! Every single day she wants me to walk to the dining room. I guess it is too much trouble for her to wheel me to the dining room in that beautiful new wheelchair that you bought for me. The service here is terrible."

Case Study #4

- Mr. C has Parkinson's disease and has fallen several times over the weekend when he forgot to use his walker while ambulating. The nurse has put him in a wheelchair and has asked you to watch him and make sure he doesn't try to get up and walk for fear that he will fall again. You know that he will become weaker every day he sits in the wheelchair without walking, and he will certainly have a decline in his functioning as a result. You approach the nurse to discuss this concern with her.

Figure 2.1 (*continued*)

Week One: Introduction to Restorative Care

The first inservice focuses on helping staff understand what restorative care involves for both older adults and care providers. Caregivers and individuals working with older adults need to understand that restorative nursing care focuses on the restoration and/or maintenance of physical function and is intended to help older adults to do things for themselves rather than being done for them. Most importantly, older adults need to be helped to focus on their abilities not disabilities. In addition, education needs to focus on helping caregivers understand that restorative care influences not only physical function but also the emotional health of older adults. When caregivers encourage physical function, older adults' overall mood, self-esteem, and quality of life will also likely be improved. For older adults with cognitive impairment and/or behavioral problems, maintaining physical function and activity is particularly important. Ultimately, the goals of restorative care are to decrease falls and incontinence, provide older adults with a sense of accomplishment, and provide opportunities for meaningful activities. If nothing else, helping older adults to know and feel that they accomplished something that day—performed an exercise program, went for a walk, or washed themselves—can have a significant psychological benefit.

This inservice also delineates for the staff what exactly is meant by restorative care activities. Examples are provided of options, including encouraging older adults to participate in their own bathing and dressing, walking to the dining room, lifting weights while waiting for meals to be served, eating as independently as possible, wearing a splint or support to facilitate function, or simply going through range of motion of joints during bathing and dressing activities. An older adult may only be able to participate in hand-over-hand type of activities (i.e., the caregiver guiding the hand of the older adult), but it is essential to recognize that this activity has important physical benefits in that the older adult is ranging his or her joints through the process. A major emphasis in this introductory inservice is on the fact that all the restorative care activities discussed can be incorporated into daily activities and should require no significant increase in caregiver time. At the end of the session, the class participants should be encouraged to brainstorm together about case examples (Table 2.4) and establish what restorative care activities could be implemented.

TABLE 2.4 Case Examples to Facilitate Discussion During Week One Inservice Training

Case 1: Mrs. Smith has had a stroke and so her balance is not perfect. She is able to get up out of the wheelchair alone and to walk with a walker as long as someone is by her side.
- What restorative care activities might you do with her?
- How could you implement this into daily activities?

Case 2: Mrs. Green has very bad arthritis and it is hard for her to hold a folk or spoon.
- What restorative care activities might you do with her?
- How could you incorporate these into daily activities?

Week Two: Restorative Care Activities

Week two provides more specific information about the how to's of restorative care. Although a review of restorative care techniques such as positioning and transferring is provided, the major focus of this educational session is on how to encourage optimal function of older adults and incorporate that into daily activities. It should be stressed to caregivers that they have the necessary knowledge and expertise to perform restorative care activities. The challenge is actually in using what they know about caregiving activities to optimize patient function, not decrease it. The inservice provides a brief overview of the different levels of assistance needed and defines and describes each level of care (i.e., independent, assistance with set up, supervision, minimum assistance, moderate assistance, and dependent). The basics of body alignment and positioning are reviewed, and the nursing assistants demonstrate how to perform these tasks themselves. Following a review of positioning, the purpose and intention of restorative care is again reviewed, focusing on how restorative care can maintain joint function, prevent deformity, build muscle strength, stimulate circulation, and build up tolerance and endurance to perform simple tasks.

A review of exercise to maintain function is then provided. Passive, active assistance, and active range of motion exercises are described and taught. These definitions are put into practical terms, and the focus is on how the exercises can be built into daily activities (Table 2.5). Passive exercises, for example, are done without the assistance of the older adult and can be carried out during bathing and dressing. Active assistance is carried out by the older adult with the help of the caregiver to encourage normal muscle function. These exercises also can be encouraged during bathing and dressing. Active range of motion exercise is done by the

TABLE 2.5 Incorporating Exercise Into Daily Activities

Example: Do these while waiting for a meal tray or at the end of bathing and dressing.

Head turns—Stand using a stable surface for balance or support.
  Look over the right shoulder; count to 5.
  Look over the left shoulder; count to 5.
  Repeat the sequence 5 times.

Airplanes—Stand using a stable surface for balance and support.
  Hold onto a stable surface with one hand.
  Hold other arm straight out to the front.
  Circle straight arm 5 times to the right and 5 times to the left.
  Repeat the sequence using the other arm.
    If able, can do both arms at the same time.

Tea pot side bends—Stand using a stable surface for balance and support.
  Hold stable surface with one hand.
  Place the other arm above your head (slightly bent).
  Bend sideways at the waist away from the raised arm.
  Return to the starting position.
  Repeat 5 times to one side, then switch arms and repeat sequence to the other side.
  Modification for those who cannot successfully reach arm above head:
    Place hand on the head to do the side bend.

Check those toes—Sit in a chair or wheelchair with feet flat on the floor.
  Lift toes up while keeping heels touching the floor.
  Count to 5.
  Lower toes to the floor.
  Repeat up to 10 times.

Hugs—Stand with stable surface within reach.
  Hold slightly bent arms horizontally out to your sides.
  Palms face each other.
  Bring arms in toward the center and give yourself a hug.
  Count to 5.
  Open arms out to the side (keeping them slightly bent).
  Repeat the sequence up to 10 times.
    A weight may be held in each hand to make the exercise a little more difficult.

Dance away the night—Sit in a chair or wheelchair.
  Begin with knees and feet as close together as possible.
  Lift the left knee about ½ inch.
  Move the left leg 5–6 inches out to the left side.
  Return to starting position.
  Repeat up to 10 times.
  Repeat the sequence using the right leg.
    An ankle weight may be used on the "working" leg to make the exercise a little harder.

Clap those hands—Place patient supine or in a semi-upright position.
  Hold arms out to sides at shoulder height.
  Palms face inward.
  Cross right arm over body to touch the left arm or hand.
  Count to 5.
  Return to starting position.
  Repeat up to 10 times.
  Switch arms and repeat up to 10 times.

older individual without any assistance from the caregiver. During active range of motion exercises, the joints are moved through a full range of motion without assistance. Joint range of motion is done when the older adult turns in bed, pushes up in bed, or transfers. Resistance exercise, in contrast to range of motion, is actively carried out by the older adult working against a force produced by another individual or with a weight. Upper extremity resistance exercise can be done easily while an older adult is waiting for a meal in the dining room or while sitting and watching television.

This inservice also goes through the use of splints and braces and the importance of correct use of these devices to promote function. During daily activities, nursing assistants must meet the needs of many older adults and often forget the importance of such devices. Ambulation techniques, the use of gait belts (as appropriate), and assistive devices are also reviewed.

Throughout the entire inservice session, it is important to stress more than the skills of performing restorative care activities. Rather, the focus should be on how to augment and encourage function, not limit it. If an older adult, for example, has a wheelchair but is ambulatory, the caregiver should encourage the older individual to walk as much as possible pushing the wheelchair. Not only does this activity increase ambulation, it also provides the older individual with an opportunity for upper extremity strengthening due to the pushing of the weight of the wheelchair.

Week Three: Restorative Care Interventions

Week three features a general overview of restorative care interventions, particularly bathing, dressing, feeding, communication, and bowel and bladder training.

As with the other inservice classes, the focus here is not on the techniques for how to perform these tasks for older individuals. Rather, the focus is on how to implement these techniques into daily activities and establish the older adult's highest potential functional ability. Table 2.6 lists the core points of this inservice, the methods to ensure restorative care success. Techniques for incorporating restorative care into all of these daily activities are addressed, and appropriate equipment and how to use it are reviewed. For example, problems with feeding and appropriate feeding equipment are identified, and the nursing assistants are given an opportunity to demonstrate how to set up and use such equipment. Simple assessment techniques, particularly for feeding are described. Examples of how to identify dysphagia and how to manage this problem are also reiterated.

Communication activities related to restorative care are discussed during this session, along with a review of the common sensory changes associated with aging. Interventions are taught to help caregivers increase older adults' participation in functional activities. Guidelines include the following: ensure that tasks are presented one at a time, ensure that tasks given to older adults proceed from simple to complex, repeat tasks, encourage activities during the older adults' peak periods of alertness, divide tasks into short (15-minute) segments, and avoid overstimulation of older adults. Recommendations for how to manage sensory changes are also considered, for example, avoiding glare and using simple lettering with high contrast such as black against white.

TABLE 2.6   Methods to Ensure Restorative Care Success

- Know the specific interventions and goals for the resident.
- Don't expect consistent performance each day. Physical and mental capability variances occur frequently and for many reasons.
- Work with the resident the same time each day.
- Include family and significant persons as much as possible to reinforce the program.
- Remove distractions from the environment.
- Adapt procedures to the resident's handicap.
- Begin working with the resident as soon as possible after admission.
- Follow the guidelines established by the restorative care nurse.
- Have the resident do as much as possible for him- or herself.
- Offer verbal cues and encouragement throughout care.
- Break tasks down into smaller steps so that the resident can complete care him- or herself.

Week three also addresses toileting as part of the restorative care program and reviews the causes of urinary incontinence and ways to institute a bladder training program, if that is appropriate for the older adult. Bowel function is likewise addressed, and a simple description of techniques to facilitate bowel function is provided. The participants are then encouraged to discuss ways to implement the skills and techniques taught in the inservice into daily activities. For example, an older adult who is able to ambulate but tends to want to sit in a wheelchair should be encouraged to increase ambulation time by walking to the bathroom every few hours. This would be an important restorative care intervention for maintaining physical function and urinary continence.

Week Four: Motivation

Week four provides an overview of motivation and reviews the many things that influence motivation in older adults. Chapter 5 discusses in depth the interventions that can be used to facilitate motivation in these individuals. It is important for administrative staff, families, and caregivers to recognize the important influence of motivation with regard to restorative care activities. When restorative care activities are not performed, it is sometimes assumed that caregivers don't know what to do or are not willing to make the effort to do it. Thus, nursing assistants and/or other caregivers are blamed for not walking or toileting individuals. In reality, the nursing assistant may have spent considerable time trying to encourage the older adult to engage in a given activity to no avail. These caregivers need to be given tools they can use to motivate these individuals to engage in the restorative care activity recommended.

After addressing motivation and ways to motivate older adults, the inservice addresses ethical concerns related to restorative care activities and concerns about persuading, (i.e., "forcing") older individuals to engage in activities they might otherwise be unwilling to perform. Many nurses, nursing assistants, and other health care providers are concerned about the rights of older adults and their ability to make choices about care activities. The choice to perform or not perform functional activities and exercise is certainly the older adult's. However, there are safety and health concerns associated with those decisions. For example, letting an older adult, develop a contracture by not ranging a joint can potentially result in significant future pain and further loss of function. Likewise, allowing an older adult to sit in one position for extended periods of time can potentially cause a pressure sore. In these scenarios, it is quite apparent that to withhold restorative care activities would be negligent on the part of the health care provider. The activities associated with restorative care are geared toward improving and maintaining function and health, and ultimately participation in these activities should be of benefit to the older adult. Attempts should be made, therefore, to encourage participation in some type of restorative care. It may be useful to negotiate with older adults and/or families as to what type of care meets their needs and goals.

Week Five: Documentation

The general restorative care recommendation (based on OBRA guidelines) is for 15 minutes at least 6 out of 7 days per week. Meeting these required recommendations allows for reimbursement of restorative activities in Medicare skilled facilities. Chapter 6 reviews in detail the documentation and reimbursement of restorative care activities. Week five training focuses on documentation of the practical ways in which restorative care can be recorded. Documentation is important, particularly in long-term care facilities, because it demonstrates the ways in which the caregivers are helping residents to obtain and maintain their highest functional level.

It is important for caregivers to understand the rational for documentation, however, no matter care setting. For example, if a facility has a large number of Medicare-covered older adults, it may be possible to capture funds related to restorative care. For all facilities, documentation would be extremely helpful to demonstrate adherence to OBRA guidelines and what staff do to prevent functional decline in residents. It would also be useful, for example, to demonstrate that although the residents have had a significant decline in function and/or an increased number of falls, they are engaging in restorative care activities daily. The increased falls may be due to increased activity, and the decline in function may be due to exacerbation of disease. These types of explanations would be very helpful for surveyors, facility administration and staff, and families.

Another important reason to document restorative care activities is to begin to consider the impact of these activities. Medicare currently requires 15 minutes of restorative care activities 6 out of 7 days per week. We do not know, however, whether or not this amount of time is sufficient. While randomized clinical trials are currently investigating the impact of restorative care, it is essential to consider the impact of these activities in real-world settings. Simple documentation of these activities could add greatly to the present state of knowledge related to restorative care.

Documentation of restorative care activities should be consistent with other documentation activities within the facility, and should not require much added time for staff. Documentation could be completed on a monthly log sheet or on a monthly calendar. Ideally, documentation should include the restorative care activity performed and the amount of time spent in the activity. In the event restorative care activities are not performed, the reason should be stated. For example, the older adult refused to participate in restorative care, the nursing assistant forgot or felt there wasn't sufficient time, or the older adult had a conflicting appointment.

Week Six: Incorporating Restorative Care Activities Into Regular Daily Care

The focus of the final week is really to reiterate how to incorporate a philosophy of care that focuses on doing *with* the older adult instead of *for*. The session encourages staff to discuss ways to address not the task that needs doing but the older adult and what he or she can do to complete the task. This could be simple such as face washing or more complex such as engaging in a daily exercise program. Restorative care can be implemented into daily care in many ways, for example, allowing older adults to turn themselves in bed, pull themselves up in bed using the rails for assistance, or stand independently without assistance from the care provider. Even if it takes a few attempts to come to a stand, for example, the activity helps to strengthen upper extremities and quadriceps. Ambulation can be incorporated into daily activities by using the walk-to-dine approach or by walking to other favorite activities. Walking can be further augmented by having the older adult push another older adult in a wheelchair. In so doing, the individual doing the pushing receives some upper extremity strengthening as well. Restorative care can be integrated into bathing activities by encouraging an older adult to bathe at his or her own speed. The environment has to be prepared for this type of self-care (e.g., appropriate bathing materials within reach). If the older adult needs cueing to continue, the caregiver can perform other tasks (e.g., make the bed or straighten the room) while cueing for the older adult to complete his or her own bathing.

Mealtime is a particularly important time for restorative care activities, and the ways that staff can encourage self-care in this area are addressed during this session. Providing and encouraging the consumption of finger foods can be of great value. Likewise, use of simple assistive devices (sippy cups, nonslide plates) to help with mealtimes, making the environment conducive to eating, and making mealtime fun can all be useful. For some older adults, combining meal and exercise time is another option. Time waiting for meal trays can be spent doing some stretching exercises and weight lifting, with weights provided at the table for that purpose.

Communication is also considered a restorative care activity, as are cognitive training and activities. This session teaches ways to talk with older adults who may have communication problems, such as expressive aphasia. The importance of talking with older adults during all care encounters is discussed, and participants are taught to encourage older adults to communicate about their families, prior work life, or special events they recall. Use of simple words and phrases and single item commands are demonstrated in this final session.

Bowel and bladder training and function generally will improve if overall physical function is increased. Functional performance is a major focus of restorative care activities, and thus bowel and bladder function may likewise improve. Combining goals related to overall physical function (e.g., increased ambulation) and improving bowel and bladder continence is ideal. If an older adult's goal is to increase ambulation, then walking to the bathroom is the optimal way in which to do that. Transferring from the commode is also a useful exercise, particularly when the older adult is encouraged to push up off the commode him- or herself instead of being lifted. Routine toileting is a very appropriate restorative care activity that can be incorporated into each older adult's daily activities, along with frequent and sufficient fluid intake.

Finally, inservice participants are reminded of the top 10 reasons to incorporate restorative care activities into their daily activities with older adults (Table 2.7), and given the opportunity to role play with established case scenarios (see case studies on last page of Figure 2.1).

ADDITIONAL INTERVENTIONS TO STRENGTHEN SELF-EFFICACY AND OUTCOME EXPECTATIONS

It is particularly important that caregivers have opportunities to strengthen their self-efficacy and outcome expectations related to performing restorative care activities. Generally, caregivers are more likely to perform restorative care activities if they have strong self-efficacy expectations about their ability to perform the activities and strong outcome expectations or beliefs about the benefits of performing the activities. With strong self-efficacy and outcome expectations, caregivers will mobilize greater effort and sustain it longer than if they harbor self-doubts and dwell on personal deficiencies when problems arise.

Verbal Persuasion

Persuasive boosts in perceived self-efficacy lead people to try hard enough to succeed, and they also promote development of skills and a sense of personal efficacy. Unfortunately, it is more difficult to instill beliefs in high personal efficacy by social persuasion

TABLE 2.7   Top 10 Reasons to Incorporate Restorative Care Into Daily Activities

It is a great way to establish a routine for the older adults.

Combining tasks makes your job easier.

Restorative care will improve older adults' functioning.

Higher functioning older adults require less strenuous care.

You have less risk of injuring yourself from lifting and pulling older adults.

You have less chance of injuring older adults from lifting and pulling.

Older adults have fewer falls and skin tears.

Family members feel more confident about the care that you provide.

Older adults feel better about themselves when they can participate in their care.

alone than it is to undermine it. Unrealistic boosts in efficacy are quickly disconfirmed by disappointing results of one's efforts. For example, a nursing assistant tries hard to get Mrs. Brown to participate in her morning care. This restorative care activity requires some additional time in morning care activities, and consequently Mrs. Brown does not get to the dining room on time for breakfast. If the nursing assistant is reprimanded for tardiness rather than praised for working on restorative care activities, her self-efficacy about her ability to incorporate restorative care activities into daily life in the facility will decrease. People who have been persuaded that they lack capabilities tend to avoid challenging activities and give up quickly in the face of difficulties. By constricting activities and undermining motivation, disbelief in one's capabilities creates its own behavioral validation. Therefore, it is essential that administration support the implementation of the restorative care program, and that all members of the team respond positively to efforts related to restorative care services.

Successful efficacy builders do more than convey positive appraisals. In addition to raising people's beliefs in their capabilities, they structure situations for them to succeed, and they avoid prematurely placing people in situations where they are likely to fail often. They develop assignments for nursing assistants to facilitate the nursing assistants' ability to incorporate restorative care activities. This might be as simple as assigning the same older adults to the same nursing assistant over time, or having a single nursing assistant care for roommates so that care oversight by the nursing assistant can be coordinated. Quite simply, the goal would be to set the individual up for successful completion of restorative care activities, and to provide positive reinforcement for the nursing assistant's efforts.

Formal meetings that focus on nursing assistants' restorative care activities are very beneficial because they capitalize on verbal encouragement. Weekly restorative care meeting is ideal because nursing assistants can report on restorative care activities and any challenges identified or successes encountered. The meeting can be run by the director of nursing, a staff nurse, the minimum data set coordinator, or an identified restorative care nurse champion within the facility. The meeting could be brief, could include walking rounds in which challenges are reviewed at the bedside (e.g., an assistive device that may not be appropriate or may not be working), or could be at staff meal-

time or change of shift so as to include as many staff members as possible.

In the home setting the family or the agency or service providing caregivers can provide verbal encouragement and ongoing assessment and feedback to caregivers. As in the institutional setting, the support and encouragement of all involved will impact ongoing restorative care behaviors. Unfortunately, in the home setting families often feel that the caregiver was hired to provide care services. Consequently, when the caregiver encourages the older adult to do activities him- or herself, families may not perceive this as a positive behavior. As in the institutional setting, it is essential that all individuals involved with the care of the older adult be included in education about restorative care activities so that they can support and believe in the benefits of this kind of care.

Vicarious Experiences

Self-efficacy expectations are also influenced by vicarious experiences or seeing other similar people successfully perform the same activity. However, certain conditions will affect the influence of vicarious experience. If the individual has not been exposed to the behavior of interest, or has had little experience with it, vicarious experience is likely to have a greater impact. In addition, the performance of others is more likely to affect personal efficacy when there are no clear guidelines for performance.

Motivating other nursing assistants and staff through the use of exemplary role models is an effective way to encourage restorative care activities. The weekly meeting with nursing assistants, or ongoing interaction in the home setting with family or supervisors, can provide a structured system in which to feature role models. Providing the role models with appropriate rewards, even if this is simply verbal recognition and praise for work well done, further augments the role modeling opportunity.

Affective States

Individuals rely in part on information from their physiological state in order to judge their abilities. Physiological indicators are especially important in relation to coping with stressors, physical accomplishments, and health functioning. Individuals evaluate their physiological state, and if it is aversive, they may avoid performing the associated behavior. For example, if a nursing assistant feels anxious about performing restorative care either because of lack of knowledge or stress to get a given assignment done, it is likely that he or she will avoid these activities. In activities involving strength and stamina, people judge their fatigue and aches and pains as signs of physical debility. Mood also affects people's judgments of their personal efficacy. Positive mood enhances perceived self-efficacy; despondent mood diminishes it.

The discussion so far has centered on efficacy-activated processes that enable people to create beneficial environments and to exercise some control over situations they encounter daily. People are partly the product of their environment. Therefore, beliefs of personal efficacy can shape the course lives take by influencing the types of activities and environments people choose. People avoid activities and situations they believe exceed their coping capabilities. But they readily undertake challenging activities and select situations they judge themselves capable of handling. By the choices they make, people cultivate different competencies, interests, and social networks that determine life courses. Any factor that influences choice behavior can profoundly affect the direction of personal development. This is because the social influences operating in selected environments continue to promote certain competencies, values, and interests long after the efficacy decisional determinant has rendered its inaugurating effect. It is not the sheer intensity of emotional and physical reactions that is important, but rather how they are perceived and interpreted. People who have a high sense of efficacy are likely to view their state of affective arousal as an energizing facilitator of performance, whereas those who are beset by self-doubts regard their arousal as a debilitator.

Physiological indicators of efficacy play an especially influential role in health functioning and in athletic and other physical activities. Nursing assistants' restorative care activities require a physical component in some circumstances, and the associated fatigue may lead to a decrease in performance of the restorative care act. For example, ambulating slowly with an older adult on the way to the dining room can, in some ways, be more fatiguing for the nursing assistant than simply pushing the individual in a wheelchair.

The best way to manage and monitor the associated sensations with restorative care is to encourage the nursing assistants, and other staff, to discuss these feelings. Feelings of frustration related to lack of administrative support for restorative care should be discussed and addressed. It may be that the nursing staff are undermining opportunities for nursing assistants to engage in restorative care by saying things like "Don't walk Mrs. M on my shift. I don't want her to fall!" Interventions that can be used to alter the interpretation of physiological feedback or help individuals cope with physiological sensations include (1) visualized mastery, which eliminates the emotional reactions to a given situation and can strengthen self-efficacy expectations and result in improvements in performance; (2) enhancement of physical status; and (3) altering the interpretation of bodily states. Understanding and discussing the sense of fatigue and boredom sometimes associated with restorative care, such as observing an older adult as he or she slowly completes a task, or walking an older adult very slowly to the dining room, can be reinterpreted as time to think, time to chat with the older adult about his or her early life, or time to share stories of your own home life. Ideas for coping with the unpleasant sensations should also be addressed during the weekly restorative care meeting.

Enactive Attainment

Enactive attainment has been described as the most influential source of efficacy information (Bandura, 1997). Repeated empirical studies have verified that actually performing an activity strengthens self-efficacy beliefs (Bandura, 1997). Performance alone, however, does not establish self-efficacy beliefs. Other factors—preconceptions of ability, the perceived difficulty of the task, the amount of effort expended, the external aid received, the situational circumstance, and the complex of past successes and failures—all impact the individual's cognitive appraisal of self-efficacy (Bandura, 1995). In light of the important influence that successful performances of restorative care activities can have, however, it is particularly useful to facilitate early restorative care successes for staff. Early success can be ensured by identifying those older adults who are most likely to participate in restorative care activities, and those for whom it is likely to be a positive experience. For example, an older adult who previously walked to the dining room would likely do so again with some encouragement. Similarly, an older adult who clearly is able to participate in some bathing activities but has been passively allowing staff to complete these tasks could be a relatively easy success if simple tasks are incorporated into morning care.

THE CHAMPION'S ROLE

No one ever said restorative care would be easy. The best way to ensure success in implementing this philosophy of care is to identify a champion and or cochampions to take the lead and facilitate the process. The champion can be a nurse or nursing assistant; someone from therapy or the activity departments; or, in the home setting, a family member or director of the home health agency. The champion needs to organize and provide inservice training, working with the staff member who coordinates inservice education. In addition, the champion should be available to help the nurses and nursing assistants determining what an older adult might or might not be able to do from a restorative care perspective and then help them establish an appropriate restorative care program for the individual. The champion might need to work with the older adult's primary care provider and therapists to establish underlying capability. Generally, however, simple baseline assessments of the older adult will provide sufficient information to determine what that individual is capable of doing.

For older adults who are functionally independent, it is important to implement a restorative care plan that maintains this optimal function. Ideally, restorative care at this level should include an exercise program. Exercise can also be incorporated into restorative care activities for all older adults, whether they are bedbound, ambulatory, or nonambulatory. Exercise programs help to optimize function, particularly when used in conjunction with ongoing performance of functional tasks.

Evaluating Older Adults for Restorative Care

A basic musculoskeletal, neurological, cognitive, affective, and functional evaluation should be performed for each older adult to determine underlying capabilities and develop an appropriate restorative plan of care. For older adults who are referred to a restorative care program after receiving traditional skilled therapy, the evaluation will already be completed and would not need to be repeated. This comprehensive evaluation serves as a baseline and can be used to follow the older adult's functional status over time. The evaluation can be easily taught to nursing assistants and can be done at intervals to monitor progress in a restorative care program to provide important information to use in completion of the minimum data set (MDS) related to the functional status of the older adult in the long-term care setting.

Instruments that can be used to augment the MDS and provide a more comprehensive evaluation of functional performance, affect, motivation, and cognition. To determine the effectiveness of the restorative care program, the instrument used must be sensitive enough to pick up small changes in the behavior you are trying to improve. For example, in an assisted living population, restorative care activities may include aerobic and resistive exercise. In this group, improvements related to restorative care activities will more likely be seen using performance measures such as the Tinetti Gait and Balance measure (Tinetti, 1986) or the timed chair rise (Gill, Williams & Tinetti, 1995). The Tinetti Gait and Balance measure provides information about the individual's gait quality and balance, and the chair rise test measures how quickly the individual can get up from a chair without using his or her arms.

Once the evaluation is completed, the champion can work with other care providers (nurses, nursing assistants, or family) to determine the activities in which the older adult will likely be able to participate. For example, an older adult who has full range of motion in an upper extremity and can follow a single-step command should be able to participate in bathing and dressing activities, even if this is done with constant verbal cues. The champion can help to develop short- and long-term goals and establish the appropriate steps for caregivers to use in helping the individual achieve those goals. Goals and methods to reach those goals should be reevaluated and updated by the champion and/or caregiver routinely (depending on the situation, once a week or once a month). This will help to ensure that success is occurring and that each older adult has the opportunity to achieve and maintain his or her highest level of functioning.

Developing the Restorative Care Plan

The champion should discuss the older adult's underlying capability with the nursing assistant or other individuals who provide direct care to the older adult. These caregivers should be encouraged to provide input in the development of short-term goals, long-term goals, and techniques to achieve those goals. The champion may seek additional input from other facility staff (e.g., nurses, therapists, activities staff), the older adult, other caregivers, and family members or other significant individuals, as appropriate. Short-term goals should coincide with each long-term goal, and stepwise progression of short-term goals should lead to accomplishing the long-term goal (Table 2.8). The short-term goals should reflect the older adult's restorative care activities and the frequency with which the activity should be performed. Each short-term goal should include nursing assistant approaches that outline the interventions to assist the older adult in meeting the goal. There may be more than one long-term goal and more than one short-term goal for each long-term goal, depending on the older adult's restorative care needs. All attempts should be made to start with short-term goals that are easy to achieve and build to more complex and challenging goals over time (Table 2.9).

Using Cues to Encourage Restorative Care Activities

Long-term goals can be written on a long-term goals form and posted in the older adult's room. Short-term goals and caregiver approaches can be written on a short-term goals form and posted in the older adult's room. These forms will provide a cue for both the older individual and the caregiver about which restorative activities should be performed. The champion can initiate a monthly calendar for the older adult that can be posted in the room next to the short-term and long-term goals forms. On the first day of each month, the champion should post a new calendar for each participating older adult.

Another option to encourage participation in restorative care activities is ongoing education of the older individual on the benefits of the restorative care activities recommended. For example, a restorative care motivational poster can be placed in the individual's room or a commonly viewed area of the home. The poster highlights the benefits of performing restorative care activities and the methods for overcoming barriers to restorative care. During daily care activities, the poster can and should be reviewed with the older individual. It serves as a reminder to perform the recommended restorative care activities and a tool to strengthen self-efficacy expectations related to

TABLE 2.8 Examples of Long- and Short-Term Goals and Nursing Assistant Approaches.

Long-Term Goal	Short-Term Goal	Nursing Assistant or Caregiver Approaches
1. The older adult will be able to walk independently to the dining room three times a day and to all activities with a rolling walker.	1. Walk ½ of the way to the dining room twice a day for meals.	Use a rolling walker. Two-person moderate assist. Rest ¼ of the way to dining room.
2. The older adult will be able to walk from the car to the house to go to her daughter's for Christmas.	2. Walk ¾ of the way to the dining room twice a day for meals.	Use a rolling walker. Two-person moderate assist. Rest ½ of the way to dining room.
	3. Walk to the dining room twice a day for . meals	Use a rolling walker. One-person moderate assist. Rest if needed.
	4. Walk to the dining room and back twice a day for meals.	Use a rolling walker. One-person standby assist. Rest if needed
	5. Walk to all activities and to the dining room and back for all meals.	Use a rolling walker. One-person standby assist. Rest when needed.

TABLE 2.9   Guidelines for Development of Goals

Component of Goal	Guidelines for Development
Goal specificity	Goals should be clear, specific, and attainable. They should explicitly state the type and amount of effort needed to attain them.
Goal challenge and proximity	Ideally, goals should be set to be moderately difficult. Relatively easy goals are not challenging enough to arouse much interest or effort, and goals set well beyond one's reach can be demotivating by undermining the individuals' efficacy beliefs.
	Pursuit of a formidable distal goal can sustain a high level of motivation if it is subdivided into subgoals that are challenging but clearly attainable through extra effort.
Goals as rewards	Remind older individuals that the reward is the ongoing process of mastery of the subgoals rather than solely in the attainment of the end goal.

restorative care. Ongoing repetition about the purpose and benefit of restorative care activities also demonstrates to the older individual that the caregiver cares enough about him or her to take the time to address restorative care activities and to encourage these activities.

Evaluating Progress

The champion should also be involved in the ongoing evaluation of the older individual with regard to restorative care activities. Ideally, a monthly evaluation of each older adult's progress toward short- and long-term goals should be done. At the time of the evaluation, the champion should seek input from all other caregivers, the individual him- or herself (as appropriate), and family members or other significant individuals as needed for an evaluation. Following this evaluation, the champion will update long- and short-term goals and caregiver approaches as needed. Changes in goals and approaches should be reflected on the goal forms and again posted in an easily visible area of the home or room of the older individual.

CONCLUSION

Motivating caregivers, including family, nurses, nursing assistants, and others who interact with older adults, is an important component of a restorative care program. Motivational interventions most likely to change behavior are driven by the theory of self-effi-

cacy. Specifically, these interventions focus on strengthening both self-efficacy and outcome expectations of the caregivers about restorative care activities. Self-efficacy expectations are the caregivers' beliefs about their ability to perform restorative care activities, especially when challenged (e.g., when tired or when there are not sufficient staff). Outcome expectations include expectations about the benefits associated with restorative care behaviors (i.e., workload will be lessened, older adults will have better quality of life). Appropriate interventions to strengthen both self-efficacy and outcome expectations include verbal persuasion, vicarious experience, affective states, and enactive attainment, that is, actually performing the activity.

REFERENCES

Allen-Burge, R., Stevens, A.B., & Burgio, L.D. (1999). Effective behavioral interventions for decreasing dementia-related challenging behavior in nursing homes. *International Journal of Geriatric Psychiatry, 14*(3), 213–228; discussion 228–232.

Almquist, E., Stein, S., Weiner, A., & Linn, M. (1981). Evaluation of continuing education for long-term care personnel: Impact upon attitudes and knowledge. *Journal of the American Geriatrics Society, 29*(3), 117–122.

Bandura, A. (1995). *Self-efficacy in changing societies.* New York: Cambridge University Press.

Bandura, A. (1997). *Self-efficacy: The exercise of control.* New York: W.H. Freeman and Company.

Beck, C., Heacock, P., Mercer, S., Walls, R., Rapp, C.G., & Vogelpohl, T. (1995). Dressing behavior in nursing home residents. *Nursing Research, 46*(3), 126–132.

Beck, C., Heacock, P., Rapp, C., & Mercer, S. (1993). Assisting cognitively impaired elders with activities of daily living. *American Journal of Alzheimer's Care and Related Disorders and Research, 8*(6), 11–20.

Beck, C., Ortigara, A., Mercer, S., & Shue, V. (1999). Enabling and empowering certified nursing assistants for quality dementia care. *International Journall of Geriatric Psychiatry, 14*(3), 197–211.

Blair, C. (1996). Combining behavior management and mutual goal setting to reduce physical dependency in nursing home residents. *Nursing Research, 44*(3), 160–164.

Bliesmer, M., & Smaylin, M. et al. (1998). The relationship between nursing staffing levels and nursing home outcomes. *Journal of Aging & Health, 10*(3), 351–372.

Bowers, B.J., Esmund, S., & Jacobson, N. Turnover reinterpreted CNAs talk about why they leave. *J Gerontol Nurs, 29*(3), 36–43.

Brown, S., Ganesan, S., & Challagalla, G. (2001). Self-efficacy as a moderator of information-seeking effectiveness. *Journal of Applied Psychology, 86*(5), 143–151.

Burgio, L., Allen-Burge, R., Roth, D., Bourgeois, M., Dijkstra, K., Gerstle, J., Jackson, E., & Bankester, L. (2001). Come talk with me: Improving communication between nursing assistants and nursing home residents during care routines. *Gerontologist, 41*(4), 449–460.

Burgio, L.D., & Burgio, K.L. (1990). Institutional staff training and management: A review of the literature and a model for geriatric nursing homes. *International Journal of Aging and Human Development, 30,* 287–302.

Cohn, M., Horgas, A., & Marsiske, M. (1990). Behavior management training for nurse aides: Is it effective? *Journal of Gerontological Nursing, 16*(11), 21–25.

Colquitt, J., LePine, J., & Noe, R. (2000). Toward an integrative theory of training motivation: A meta-analytic path analysis of 20 years of research. *Journal of Applied Psychology, 85*(5), 678–707.

Feuerberg, M. (2001). Appropriateness of minimum nurse staffing ratios in nursing homes: Overview of phase II report: Background, study approach, findings, and conclusions. Centers for Medicare and Medicaid Services Baltimore, Maryland and www.ahepv.gov/news/ulp/tcwork/ulptewy.htm, 2004.

Fleishell, A., & Resnick, B. (1999). *Stayin alive: Developing and implementing a restorative care nursing program.* Laurel, MD: Joanne Wilson's Gerontological Nursing Ventures.

Gibson, C. (2001). Me and us: Differential relationships among goal-setting training, efficacy and effectiveness at the individual and team level. *Journal of Organizational Behavior, 22*(7), 789–808.

Gill, T., Williams, C., & Tinetti, M. (1995). Assessing risk for the onset of functional dependence among older adults: The role of physical performance. *Journal of the American Geriatrics Society, 43*(6), 603–609.

Gonge, H., Jensen, L., & Bonde, J. (2002). Are psychosocial factors associated with low-back pain among nursing personnel? *Work & Stress, 16*(1), 79–87.

Grabois, M., & Coumbus, D. (1975). Rehabilitation care course for paraprofessional personnel. *Archives of Physical Medicine & Rehabilitation, 56*(3), 122–125.

Jex, S., Bliese, P., Buzzell, S., & Primeau, J. (2001). The impact of self-efficacy on stressor-strain relations: Coping style as an explanatory mechanism. *Journal of Applied Psychology, 86*(3), 401–409.

Karl, K., Olerykelly, A., & Martocchio, J. (1993). The impact of feedback and self-efficacy on performance in training. *Journal of Organizational Behavior, 14*(4), 379–394.

Kopiec, K. (2000). The work experiences of certified nursing assistants in New Hampshire: Report submitted to the New Hampshire community loan fund. Retrieved August 1, 2003. from http://www.directcareclearinghouse.org/download/work_exp_cnas_nh.pdf

Lekan-Rutledge, D., Palmer, M.H., & Belyea, M. (1998). In their own words: Nursing assistants' perceptions of barriers to implementation of prompted voiding in long-term care. *Gerontologist, 38*(3), 370–378.

Lipscomb, J., Trinkoff, A., Geiger-Brown, J., & Brady, B. (2002). Work-schedule characteristics and reported musculoskeletal disorders of registered nurses. *Scandanavian Journal of Work Environmental Health, 28*(6), 394–401.

Martocchio, J. (1994). Effects of conceptions of ability on anxiety, self-efficacy, and learning in-training. *Journal of Applied Psychology, 79*(6), 819–825.

Morgan, D.G., Semchuk, K.M., Stewart, N.J., D'Arcy, C. (2002). Rural families caring for a relative with dementia: barriers to use of formal services. *Soc Sci Med, 55*(7), 1129–1142.

Morris, J.N., Fiatarone, M., Kiely, D.K., Belleville-Taylor, P., Murphy, K., Littehale, S., Ooi, W.L., O'Neill, E., & Doyle, N. (1999). Nursing rehabilitation and exercise strategies in the nursing home. *Journal of Gerontology Series A Medical Sciences, 54A,* M494–M500.

National Citizens' Coalition for Nursing Home Reform. (2001). The nurse staffing crisis in nursing homes. Retrieved from http://nccnhr.news.com/govpolicy/51_162_701.cfm

Ootim, B. (1998). Self-esteem. *Nursing Management, 4*(10), 24–25.

Parsons, S., Simmons, W., Penn, K., & Furlough, M. (2003). Determinants of satisfaction and turnover among nursing assistants: The results of a statewide survey. *Journal of Gerontological Nursing, 21,* 51–56.

Randle, J. (2001). The effect of a 3-year pre-registration training course on students' self-esteem. *Journal of Clinical Nursing, 10*(2), 293–300.

Remsburg, R., Palmer, M.H., Langford, A.M., & Mendelson, G. (1999). Staff compliance with and ratings of effectiveness of a prompted voiding program in a long-term care facility. *Journal of Wound Ostomy Continence Nursing, 26*(5), 261–269.

Resnick, B., & Fleishell, A. (1999). Restoring quality of life. *Advance for Nurses, 1,* 10–12.

Resnick, B., & Simpson, M. (2003). Restorative care nursing activities: Pilot testing self-efficacy and outcome expectation measures. *Geriatric Nursing, 24*(2), 82–86.

Rheaume, A. (2003). The changing division of labor between nurses and nursing assistants in New Brunswick. *Journal of Advanced Nursing, 41*(5), 435–443.

Sahyoun, N., Pratt, L., Lentzner, H., Dey, A., & Robinson, K. (2001). The challenging profile of nursing home residents: 1985–1997. *Aging Trends, 4.* Hyattsville, Maryland: National Center for Health Statistics.

Salas, E., & Cannon-Bowers, J. (2001). The science of training: A decade of progress. *Annual Reviews Psychology, 52,* 471–499.

Schirm, V., Albanese, T., Garland, T. N., Gibson, G., & Blackmon, D. J. (2000). Caregiving in nursing homes: views of licensed nurses and nursing assistants. *Clin Nurs Res, 9*(3), 280–297.

Schnelle, J., Cruise, P., Rahman, A., & Ouslander, J. (1998). Developing rehabilitative behavioral interventions for long-term care: Technology transfer, acceptance and maintenance issues. *Journal of the American Geriatrics Society, 46,* 771–777.

Sinervo, T. (Ed.). (2000). *Work in care for the elderly: Combining theories of job design, stress, information processing and organizational cultures.* Academic dissertation. Saarijarvi, Finland: Gummerus Printing.

Stevens, A.B., Burgio, L.D., Bailey, E., Burgio, K.L., Paul, P., Capilouto, E., Nicovich, P., & Hale, G. (1998). Teaching and maintaining behavior management skills with nursing assistants in a nursing home. *Gerontologist, 38*(3), 379–384.

Tinetti, M. (1986). Performance oriented assessment of mobility problems in elderly patients. *Journal of the American Geriatrics Society, 34,* 199–206.

Trinkoff, A., Lipscomb, J., Geiger-Brown, J., Storr, C., & Brady, B. (2003). Perceived physical demands and reported musculoskeletal problems in registered nurses. *American Journal of Preventative Medicine, 24*(3), 270–275.

Vogelpohl, T. S., Beck, C. K., Heacock, P., & Mercer, S. O. (1996). "I can do it!" Dressing: promoting independence through individualized strategies. *J Gerontol Nurs, 22*(3), 39–42.

Wolfe, S., Nordstrom, C., & Williams, K. (1998). The effects of enhancing self-efficacy prior to job training. *Journal of Social Behavior & Personality, 13*(4), 633–651.

CHAPTER 3

Evaluating the Older Adult for Restorative Care

Marianne Shaughnessy and Barbara Resnick

A comprehensive evaluation is a necessary component of initiating restorative care services for the older adult. Well-documented baseline evaluation provides information needed for designing a program appropriate for the particular needs of an older adult and serves as a benchmark to evaluate progress over time. It is particularly essential to perform a comprehensive history and a musculoskeletal, neurological, cognitive, affective, and functional examination of the older adult to determine underlying capabilities. For older adults who are referred to a restorative care program after receiving traditional skilled therapy, a similar evaluation would already have been completed and can be used for restorative care planning and to follow the older adult's functional status over time.

Obtaining an accurate history and physical is a skill when working with all adults, but it is particularly challenging when working with older adults. These challenges are due to normal changes that occur with aging, the tendency for diseases to present in an atypical fashion, their long medical histories, and common communication problems because of sensory changes, aphasia, or cognitive impairment.

When beginning an evaluation of an older adult, a key point to remember is to allow sufficient time to do a comprehensive history and physical. It may be appropriate, if the patient has a long and complicated past medical history or fatigues easily, to break up the history and physical examination to separate visits, scheduling up to an hour for each visit. Increased time may be needed to help these individuals into the examination room and with dressing and undressing, and to repeat questions and confirm answers. Time spent obtaining accurate information about the older adult's medical history, disease processes, functional status,

and functional desires yields benefits in the design of an appropriate, goal-oriented plan of restorative care.

TAKING THE HISTORY

The format for history taking with older patients is similar to that with younger patients. That is, the history should ideally include chief complaint, history of present illness, past history, medication use, social history, family history, and a review of systems. However, some liberalization of the traditional interpretation of these components of the history is necessary to be most relevant to the needs of the older adult.

Traditionally the adult patient is the primary source of information for the history. However, because of cognitive changes or a lack of interest or knowledge about their medical problems, many older adults are unable to provide comprehensive medical information. Attempt to use lay terminology that is culturally relevant to elicit more comprehensive information (e.g., "sugar" for diabetes). When working with these individuals, it may be necessary to get information from prior medical records (records from an acute care hospital stay or an outpatient or nursing home chart) and/or from family, friends, and staff. The choice to have a family member present during the history and examination should be based on the patient's wishes. If a family member is present during the exam, it should be made clear that the patient is to answer the questions when possible, not the relative. The relative can help at the end of the history for clarification and augmentation of findings.

Even patients with known cognitive impairment, or those noted to be unreliable in terms of their ability to provide information for the history, should be given an opportunity to answer questions and describe their symptoms. It is, however, essential to evaluate the individual's cognitive status to determine his or her ability to provide reliable health information. Even when there is severe dementia, questions regarding current symptoms and functional goals may still yield useful information, and it is important to establish a caring relationship by listening to these individuals. To establish an overall sense of the patient's cognitive status quickly, begin the history taking with questions that focus on orientation and verifiable medical history. For example, ask questions about time and place orientation, reasons for the visit, previous health care contacts, biographical data, and medication use.

Though your focus will be on evaluation of the patient's current capabilities for restorative care services, the history should begin with a query about current problems that should be addressed as soon as possible. Resolution of minor acute medical problems or optimal management of chronic problems will facilitate implementation of restorative care plans. A chief complaint and history of present illness should be documented, as with any patient. Older adults, particularly those with cognitive impairment, may have some difficulty remembering chronology of events or describing symptoms completely. Using open-ended questions and providing choices of adjectives may help the patient describe symptoms and illness more completely. Table 3.1 provides a comprehensive checklist to use to determine if any interventions are needed prior to implementing specific restorative care activities (e.g., symptoms of pain or shortness of breath that are not stable for that individual). The checklist can also be used to help focus the development of the restorative care plan. Recognizing, for example, that an individual is not independent with eating could be the initial focus of the restorative care program. Likewise, significant problems with musculoskeletal pain might lead to focusing a restorative care program on range of motion and pool exercises to augment function and decrease pain. This baseline evaluation will also be useful for the ongoing evaluation of the resident once restorative care has been implemented.

Medications

It is essential to carefully review and evaluate every medication the older individual is taking, both pre-

scribed and over the counter. Do not forget to consider vitamins, minerals, herbs, laxatives, sleeping pills, and cold preparations as these may interact with other medications and have an impact on function and performance. When reviewing medication, it is a good time to also consider the use of nicotine, alcohol, and illicit drugs. Older adults may be asked how much alcohol they drink, rather than if they drink, presenting a nonjudgmental approach by the examiner. Carefully document the individual's use of these substances and follow up or refer, as appropriate.

Past Medical History

It is not uncommon for older adults to have an extensive past medical history. Begin by asking the older patient about known medical problems and/or by reviewing is already documented in the history. When asking questions, provide prompts such as "Do you remember being told you had a problem with your heart, lungs, stomach, liver, or kidneys?" Next ask about specific diseases such as diabetes, hypertension, depression, or cancer. Another way to prompt memory for some of these problems is to ask about past hospitalizations and the reason for those hospitalizations. Do not focus on childhood illnesses, with the exception of asking about any childhood illness that kept them in bed or out of school for an extended period of time (e.g., rheumatic fever). Reviewing medications is another useful way to stimulate the older adult to recall prior diagnoses and medical problems. Taking the time to establish a medical history that is as comprehensive as possible is essential to prevent recurrence of prior problems, and also to help understand functional changes they may have occurred.

Past Surgical History

With past surgical history, it may be necessary to prompt older patients' memory with questions about common surgeries that occur with age such as cataracts, joint replacements, or removal of skin lesions. It is also necessary to ask specifically about the removal of organs such as the gallbladder, appendix, uterus, or prostate. When doing the physical exam, confirm any scars that are evident with the surgical

TABLE 3.1   Checklist for Restorative Care Evaluation

Clincial Focus	Independent	Semidependent	Totally Dependent
Function performance 　Mobility 　Bathing 　Dressing 　Eating 　Toileting			
	Yes	No	Stable
Medications 　Psychotropics* 　Alcohol 　Nicotine 　Narcotics			
Past medical history 　Orthopedic problems 　Cognitive problems 　Neurological problems 　Pulmonary problems requiring oxygen use			
Social supports 　Family involved 　Friends involved 　Participates in group activities			
Current symptoms/physical abnormalities 　Sensory 　Cardiovascular 　Respiratory 　Gastrointestinal 　Urinary 　Musculoskeletal 　Neurological 　Integumentary 　Cognitive/Affective			
Screening for physical activity	Done	Not Needed	

*Pyschotropics include antidepressants, anxiolytics, antiseizure medications, and sedative hypnotics.

history given, and question the patient about any unexplained scars noted.

Social History

Social information is relevant for the older patient in any setting because it is important to understand what supports the older individual has to help with activities of daily living and instrumental activities of daily living. Determining if the individual has private nursing assistants, family, friends, or neighbors who help with these activities or provide support in any way is useful. If the individual lives in the home setting, information about the community at large may be useful. In any care setting, look for the presence and condition of any stairs, the distances needed to walk to the bathroom, the accessibility of the kitchen, and the activities the individual currently needs assistance with (grocery shopping, cooking, cleaning, laundry). Observe also for safe areas in which distance ambulation can occur. Explore all potential social supports with the patient, and determine what type of interaction they have with the patient (phone calls or visits). The social support network may be useful in helping to implement aspects of the restorative care plan and/or may be important sources of goals or rewards. For example, some people can be motivated to bathe and dress to be ready for a visit. Specific assessment tools such as the MOS Social Support Survey (http://www. rand.org/health/surveys/mos.descrip.html) or the Social Support for Exercise Scale (Sallis et al., 1985) may be useful for assessing the support the individual has available.

Nutritional History

A nutritional history is best obtained by asking the older patient and/or caregivers to describe a typical 24-hour diet and pattern of weight during recent years. Also explore shopping and food preparation habits and food preferences and concerns. In particular, older adults should be asked about an involuntary weight change. Weight loss of 5 pounds in 6 months or less is indicative of protein-energy malnutrition (Daly & Adelman, 2000).

Functional Assessment

The most critical component of the history in evaluating older adults for restorative care activities is func-

TABLE 3.2 List of Functional Scales

The PULSES Profile (Moskowitz, 1957).

Index of Independence in Activities of Daily Living (ADL) (Katz, Ford, & Moskowitz, 1963).

The Barthel Index (Mahoney & Barthel, 1965).

The Kenny Self-Care Evaluation (Schoening et al., 1965; Schoening & Iverson, 1968).

The Physical Self-Maintenance Scale (Lawton & Brody, 1969).

The Medical Outcomes Study Physical Functioning Measure (Stewart & Kamburg, 1992).

A Rapid Disability Rating Scale (Linn & Linn, 1982).

The Dartmouth COOP Functional Health Assessment Charts (Nelson et al., 1996).

The Functional Status Index (Jette & Deniston, 1978; Jette, 1980).

The Edmonton Functional Assessment Tool (Kaasa et al., 1997).

The Self-Evaluation of Life Function Scale (Linn, 1982).

The Functional Activities Questionnaire (Pfeffer, 1982; Pfeffer et al., 1984).

The Lambeth Disability Screening Questionnaire (Patrick, Darby, & Green, 1981).

Stanford Health Assessment Questionnaire (Fries, Spitz, & Young, 1982).

FIM™ Instrument (Hamilton et al., 1987).

TABLE 3.3   Katz Index of ADLs

1. Bathing (sponge, shower, or tub)
   I: recieves no assistance (gets in and out of the tub)
   A: receives assistance in bathing only one part of the body
   D: receives assistance in bathing more than one part of the body
2. Dressing
   I: gets clothes and gets completely dressed without assistance
   A: gets clothes and gets dressed without assistance except in tying shoes
   D: receives assistance in getting clothes or in getting dressed or stays partly or completely undressed
3. Toileting
   I: goes to toilet room, cleans self, and manages clothes without assistance (may use an assistive device)
   A: receives assistance in going to the toilet room, in cleaning self or managing clothes, or in emptying a bedpan
   D: doesn't go to toilet room for elimination
4. Transfer
   I: moves in and out of bed as well as in and out of chair without assistance (may use assistive device)
   A: moves in and out of bed or chair with assistance
   D: doesn't get out of bed
5. Continence
   I: controls urination and bowel movements independently
   A: has occasional accidents
   D: supervision helps keep urine or bowel control; uses catheter or is incontinent
6. Feeding
   I: feeds self without assistance
   A: feeds self except for getting assistance in cutting meat or buttering bread
   D: receives assistance in feeding or is fed partly or completely by using tubes or intravenous fluids

Abbreviations: I = independent; A = assistance; and D = dependent

tional performance. Functional evaluations should include activities of daily living (ADLs) such as eating, bathing, dressing, transferring, toileting, and ambulation. Instrumental activities of daily living (IADLs) are higher level activities, such as those required for living in the community, and include activities such as taking medications, paying bills, using the telephone, and using public transportation. Standardized functional status instruments are very useful in obtaining this baseline information and following progress over time. Many such instruments are available, and the decision to use one over the other may depend on the population (Table 3.2). For example, the Katz Index (Katz, Ford, & Moskowitz, 1963) for both ADLs and IADLs (Tables 3.3 and 3.4) is a basic measure that helps describe the patient as either dependent, semidependent, or independent in activities of daily living. It will not, however, identify small changes in the individual over time. The Barthel Index (Mahoney & Barthel, 1965) provides a graduated scale of dependence to independence for each activity and is more sensitive to incremental changes in functional status over time (Table 3.5). The items on the functional measures serve as a guide to help in the assessment of what the patient can perform functionally and/or what assistance is needed.

A careful functional status examination provides the basis for identifying *capabilities* versus what the individual might actually be doing. A brief discussion should follow this assessment regarding functional goals or desired activities the individual would like to perform so that goals can be appropriately chosen. It is important to distinguish what the health care provider,

TABLE 3.4 Instrumental Activities of Daily Living (IADLs)

1. Telephone
   I: able to look up numbers, dial, and receive and make calls without help
   A: able to answer phone or dial operator in an emergency, but needs special phone or help in getting number or dialing
   D: unable to use the telephone
2. Traveling
   I: able to drive own care or travel alone on bus or taxi
   A: able to travel but not alone
   D: unable to travel
3. Shopping
   I: able to take care of all shopping with transportation provided
   A: able to shop but not alone
   D: unable to shop
4. Preparing meals
   I: able to plan and cook full meals
   A: able to prepare light foods, but unable to cook full meals alone
   D: unable to prepare any meals
5. Housework
   I: able to do heavy housework (scrub floors)
   A: able to do light housework, but needs help with heavy tasks
   D: unable to do any housework
6. Medication
   I: able to take medications in the right dose at the right time
   A: able to take medications, but needs reminding or someone to prepare it
   D: unable to take medications
7. Money
   I: able to manage buying needs, write checks, pay bills
   A: able to manage daily buying needs, but needs help managing checkbook and paying bills
   D: unable to manage money

Abbreviations: I = independent; A = assistance; and D = dependent

TABLE 3.5 Barthel Index

Level of Care	Intact	Limited	Helper	Null
Self-Care				
Feed	10( )	5( )	3( )	3( )
Dress UE	5( )	5( )	3( )	0( )
Dress LE	5( )	5( )	2( )	0( )
Don brace	0( )	0( )	–2( )	0( )
Grooming	5( )	5( )	0( )	0( )
Wash	4( )	4( )	0( )	0( )
Perineum	4( )	4( )	2( )	0( )
	[Complete Voluntary]	[Urgency/ Appliance]	[Some help needed]	[Frequent accidents]
Sphincters				
Bladder	10( )	10( )	5( )	0( )
Bowel	10( )	10( )	5( )	0( )
	[Easy/No device]	[With difficulty or uses device]	[Some help]	[Dependent]
Mobility Transfer:				
Chair	15( )	15( )	7( )	0( )
Toilet	6( )	5( )	3( )	0( )
Tub	1( )	1( )	0( )	0( )
Walk 50 yds	15( )	15( )	10( )	0( )
Stairs	10( )	10( )	5( )	0( )
W/C 50 yds	15( )	5( )	0( )	0( )none

in collaboration with the entire health care team, perceives the individual to be capable of doing versus what the individual actually does on a daily basis. The individual and/or family may have unrealistic expectations about capability or the patient may be allowing caregivers to perform tasks that he or she is actually able to perform. Combining the functional assessment with the musculoskeletal and neurological evaluation described below will help to differentiate underlying capability from actual performance.

SYSTEMS REVIEW

In addition to obtaining a good history, it is helpful to do a current review of all systems to evaluate what signs and symptoms the patient or caregivers identify. The review of systems with older adults should focus on problems that are particularly prevalent in this population, specifically, a change in cognition, urinary or bowel incontinence, falls, immobility, insomnia, dysphagia, and sensory changes. Positive responses to any of these questions can be a useful starting point to a more comprehensive evaluation of the problem and the identification of a more serious underlying problem.

Sensory Changes

Changes in vision and hearing have the potential to dramatically impact restorative care efforts and must be carefully investigated and documented. A number of normal age changes in vision and common problems experienced by older patients (cataracts, macular degeneration, and glaucoma) influence sensory function. Normal age changes include increased sensitivity to glare and decreases in visual acuity, elasticity of the lens, peripheral vision, color intensity (specifically for the shades of blue, green, and purple), night vision and accommodation to changes in lighting, tear production and viscosity, depth perception, and near vision (presbyopia). In light of all these changes, it is essential to ask older adults about visual changes and their ability to read normal print and/or large print materials. Dry eyes and tearing due to blocked tear ducts are also very common in older adults and should be specifically explored.

Similarly, age-related changes in the ear impact hearing. The tympanic membrane becomes thicker, more fixed, and less translucent and loses its luster. The cerumen is thicker, drier, and harder. In the cochlea, hair cells, neurons, supporting cells, ganglion cells, and fibers all decrease. These cochlear changes alter hearing and balance. Ask the older patient specifically about hearing changes, any prior history of hearing evaluations, and if their ears have been checked for wax accumulation, which is the most common cause of hearing loss. Tinnitus is a common complaint and is often described as a loud or muted ringing in the ear or head. Tinnitus can be related to presbycusis (sensorineural hearing loss) due to the deterioration of the hair cells in the chochlea and deterioration of the central auditory pathways in the brain.

Cardiovascular Review

Unfortunately, the presentation of cardiovascular disease in older adults is often not associated with the typical signs and symptoms found in younger individuals. For example, an older adult with atrial fibrillation may have no symptoms at all or may complain vaguely of just not feeling right (Resnick, 1999). Ask the patient about any subtle changes in function or activity, which may be related to progressive cardiovascular disease. Explore in particular whether the indi- vidual notes any shortness of breath, swelling in the feet or hands, dizziness, cough, or orthopnea. Any positive findings on the cardiac review should be evaluated and potential problems treated prior to instituting a restorative care plan.

Respiratory Review

Respiratory disorders are common in older adults and the review of systems should focus on exploring with these individuals the associated symptoms of these diseases, such as shortness of breath and cough. Patients may describe themselves as having breathing difficulties or having trouble getting a deep breath or sufficient air. As in the cardiac review of systems, ask the older patients about when dyspnea occurs (i.e., with how much exertion) by having them consider their performance of specific activities. Also explore for any change in the ability to perform usual activities. Cough is a common pulmonary complaint, and patients should be asked when the cough occurs and the existence, color, amount, and consistency of any sputum. If there is a new onset cough, determine whether the patient started any new medications or was exposed to a change in environment.

Gastrointestinal Review

Constipation is one of the most common digestive complaints in older adults and may have dangerous complications, including acute changes in cognition, urinary retention, urinary incontinence, and fecal impaction. Chronic constipation, if left untreated, can lead to significant morbidity and, rarely, mortality in older adults. Fecal impaction from constipation can result in intestinal obstruction, ulceration, and urinary problems. Chronic straining to defecate can cause adverse effects on cerebral, coronary, and peripheral vascular circulation. Constipation must be considered a serious problem for older adults, and one that is deserving of a comprehensive evaluation and management plan.

Acute abdominal pain may reflect a critical gastrointestinal problem in older adults. Recognition and diagnosis of acute abdominal problems in older adults is especially important because delay in treatment doubles the risk of mortality. The challenge in diagnosis is greatest in these individuals because of their inability to provide subjective reports of pain and because they are likely not to manifest a fever or leukocytosis with an abdominal infection (Parker, Vukov, & Wollan, 1996). Acute abdominal problems in older adults include those associated with obstruction, inflammation, ischemia/vascular disorders, systemic disorders, and primary peritoneal disease. Unfortunately, a worsening of cognitive and functional status may be the only presenting symptom in older adults.

The incidence of colorectal cancers is increased in older adults (Mariotto, et at., 2003). To identify these malignancies early, therefore, the review of the gastrointestinal system should focus on changes in bowel habits, evidence of a change in color of the stool or blood in the stool, weight loss, decreased appetite, and abdominal distension or discomfort. Hemorrhoids are also common, and questioning about painful bowel movements, pain when sitting, and consistency of the stool are useful. This is also a good time to encourage older adults to have a fecal occult blood test as a screening for bowel cancer.

Gastroesophageal reflux disease is another very prevalent gastrointestinal problem in older adults. Symptoms of reflux may be typical burning and indigestion within 30 minutes of eating, with these symptoms being aggravated if the individual reclines or bends over. Patients may also complain of chest pain and heaviness, gas, increased saliva, difficulty swallowing, a sore throat, or hoarseness. The challenge in working with older adults is to differentiate these symptoms from those of cardiac disease, which is sometimes only done by response to specific treatments.

Genitourinary Review

Urinary incontinence is often not reported by older adults because they consider it to be a normal age change and have low expectations of benefit from treatment. When evaluating incontinence, ask older adults if they have trouble getting to the bathroom on time, if they need to wear a pad, and how many times a day they have to change the pad. Table 3.6 describes the different types of urinary incontinence and provides useful information for determining the underlying cause of incontinence.

If the patient has complaints of urinary incontinence, get as much information as possible to determine what type of incontinence may be present. To distinguish the cause, questioning should focus on what time of the day the incontinence occurs, and what type of activity exacerbates the incontinence. For example, ask the patient if the incontinence occurs with coughing or sneezing or if it occurs on the way to the bathroom or at night. The number of pads worn helps to determine the degree of the incontinence, although the patient should also be asked how much the

TABLE 3.6   Urinary Incontinence

Type of Incontinence	Definition	Pathophysiology	Signs and Symptoms
Stress	An involuntary loss of urine due to urethral sphincter failure with increases in intrabdominal pressure	Usually caused from weakness and laxity of pelvic floor musculature or bladder outlet weakness Urethral hypermobility	Urine lost during coughing, sneezing, laughing
Urge	Leakage of urine because of inability to delay voiding after sensation of bladder fullness perceived	Associated with detrusor hyperactivity, central nervous system disorders, or local genitourinary conditions	Urine lost on the way to the bathroom or as soon as the urge to void felt
Overflow	Leakage of urine resulting from mechanical forces on an overdistended bladder	Results from mechanical obstruction or an acontractile bladder	Variety of symptoms, including frequent or constant dribbling and increased incontinence at night Frequency and urgency also noted
Functional	Leakage of urine associated with inability to get to the toilet because of cognitive and/or physical functioning	Cognitive and physical functional impairment	Patient aware of the need to void but urine lost on the way to the bathroom

incontinence interferes with his or her ability (or desire) to do daily activities and/or engage in social activities. During the review of systems, the practitioner needs to begin to identify any potential reversible causes of incontinence.

Prostate disorders in an older man may cause urinary incontinence, although the existence of other symptoms is also possible. Ask the male patient specifically about frequent urination, hesitancy, weak or intermittent stream, and a sensation of incomplete emptying of the bladder and dribbling after voiding.

The incidences of urinary tract infections also increase with age, particularly in postmenopausal women. Older adults may not necessarily present with the typical dysuria, urgency, frequency, lower abdominal pain, and fever. Rather, they may report new-onset incontinence, loss of appetite, vomiting, falls, nocturia, difficulty urinating, or behavioral and cognitive changes. The practitioner should ask about these symptoms to help identify the possibility of a urinary tract infection.

MUSCULOSKELETAL AND NEUROLOGICAL REVIEW

In the evaluation of older adults for restorative care services, special attention must be paid to musculoskeletal and neurological dysfunction. Older adults tend to under-report musculoskeletal symptoms because they believe these are due to aging or because they do not want any further treatment. Osteoarthritis is the most common joint disease in older adults, affecting over 80% of individuals 65 years of age and older (Nesher & Moore, 1994). Older patients should be asked about pain, stiffness, joint enlargement, decreased range of motion, and functional changes. Similarly, the incidence of rheumatoid arthritis increases in older adults, and appropriate diagnosis is sometimes difficult because of the presence of both osteoarthritis and rheumatoid arthritis. The clinician therefore needs to be familiar with the classic signs and symptoms of both osteoarthritis and rheumatoid arthritis to make this differentiation (Table 3.7).

Other diagnoses commonly seen in older adults that may affect musculoskeletal function include gout, polymyalgia rheumatica, and osteoporosis. Assessment for these disorders should include specific questions about joint swelling, range of motion, stiffness, fractures, loss of height, and bone pain.

Although falls may be caused by a number of factors, questions about falls are appropriate when addressing the musculoskeletal system. Table 3.8 provides a quick guide for the evaluation of falls and can help differentiate if the fall is due to gait or balance disorders or another underlying disorder for which the patient should be evaluated and treated.

Changes in the neurological system, due either to normal changes or disease, can result in subtle to severe changes in an older adult in balance, mobility, coordination, sensory interpretations, level of consciousness, intellectual performance, personality,

TABLE 3.7 Differences in Signs and Symptoms Between Osteoarthritis and Rheumatoid Arthritis

	Osteoarthritis	Rheumatoid Arthritis
Joint characteristics	Asymmetrical involvement Cool to touch Crepitus Mono- or polyarticular Polyarticular	Symmetrical involvement Boggy joints that may be warm, red, and tender
Joints involved	Distal and proximal interphalanges Weight-bearing joints Spine	Metacarpals, metatarsals, and wrists
Pain	Morning stiffness lasting less than an hour Pain relieved with ice, exercise	Morning stiffness lasting longer than 1 hour Pain at rest
Systemic involvement	None	Fatigue Anorexia Malaise Depression

TABLE 3.8   Evaluation of Falls

Patient name: _____ Age: __ Gender: ___ Date: _____

Risk factors for subsequent falls

1. History of previous falls
   a. Yes
   b. No
2. Medications:
   a. Four or more prescriptions
   b. New prescription in the last 2 weeks
   c. Use of any of the following medications: tranquilizers, sleeping pills, antidepressants, cardiac medications, antidiabetic agents
3. Known gait problem or muscular weakness
   a. Yes
   b. No
4. Dizziness, vertigo, or loss of consciousness at time of fall
   a. Yes
   b. No
5. Visual changes
   a. Yes
   b. No
6. Environmental problems
   a. Clutter
   b. Lighting
   c. Uneven flooring
   d. Footwear/lack of footwear
   e. Inappropriate assistive device
7. Major illnesses
   a. Neurological: Parkinson's disease, stroke, dementia
   b. Musculoskeletal: arthritis, contracture, fracture
   c. Cardiac: hypotension, arrhythmia, acute infarct
   d. New acute illness: infection
   e. Other
8. Additional questions:
   a. What happened at the time of the fall, i.e., what was the patient doing? _____
   _____
   _____
   b. Were any injuries associated with the fall?
      1. Laceration
      2. Sprain/strain
      3. Fracture
      4. Persistent pain
      5. Head trauma
      6. Other
   c. How has course been since the fall?
      1. Associated fear of falling?
      2. Change in function?
      3. Change in cognition?
   d. Is the patient able to carry on usual activities, and if not who is available to help with usual activities? _____
   _____
   _____

communication, comprehension, emotional responses, and thoughts. Strokes are the most common neurological problem in older adults, and patients should be asked about possible signs and symptoms of a stroke (Table 3.9).

Parkinson's disease is the most common extrapyramidal movement disorder seen in older adults. Parkinson's disease is characterized by decreased voluntary movement, increased involuntary movements (tremor), impaired muscle tone, and impaired postural reflexes, and a large number of signs and symptoms result from these problems (Table 3.10). All older adults should be asked about these signs and symptoms. It is especially important to ask patients who have a known history of Parkinson's disease whether they are currently experiencing symptoms related to the Parkinson's disease, as this may influence treatment.

Vertigo is a common problem in older adults, and diagnosis is based mainly on clinical symptoms. Ask patients specifically about spatial disorientation, characterized as a sensation of rotational movement involving the individual and or the surroundings. Older adults can be asked if they feel as if the room is spin-

TABLE 3.9   Signs and Symptoms of Stroke

Vessel Involved	Signs and Symptoms
Internal carotid artery	Hemiplegia
	Aphasia (expressive and receptive)
	Visual changes
	Neglect
	Agnosia
	Apraxia
Middle cerebral artery	Hemiplegia
	Aphasia (expressive)
	Visual changes
	Apraxia
	Decreased attention
Anterior cerebral artery	Hemiparesis
	Emotional lability
	Aphasia (expressive)
	Cognitive changes
	Incontinence
Posterior cerebral artery	Decreased sensation and dysethesias
	Neglect
	Visual changes
	Decreased sensory attention
Vertebrobasilar	Quadriplegia
	Loss of brain stem reflexes
	Coma

TABLE 3.10 Signs and Symptoms of Parkinson's Disease

Decreased strength
Difficulty walking, with shuffling
Falls
Difficulty turning over in bed
Increased fatigue and lethargy
Slowness of movement
Decreased facial expression
Increased time needed for any activity (bathing, dressing, ambulation)
Changes in handwriting
Changes in voice quality
Difficulty swallowing
Changes in memory
Weight loss
Pill rolling tremor at rest
Drooling

ning, or if they feel as if they are spinning. Finally, when there is a complaint of vertigo or dizziness, these individuals should be asked about associated symptoms of nausea, vomiting, hearing loss, or tinnitus.

The incidences of seizures significantly increases in individuals over the age of 65 due to an increase in strokes, tumors, subdural hematomas, metabolic disorders, and dementia, as well as in response to medications. Older adults should be asked not only whether they have a known history of seizures but also whether they have noted any episodes of repetitive shaking or muscle contractions, brief lapses of consciousness, or any abnormal sensations that they can associate with a seizure.

INTEGUMENTARY REVIEW

There are many age-related changes in the skin, whether due to age and/or the environment, and they often result in uncomfortable symptoms such as pruritus. Ask older adults specifically about their skin care practices, such as frequency of bathing and type of soap used, sun exposure, use of creams or cosmetics, radiation exposure, and professional work area (even if they are retired) because these factors might influence current skin condition. Ask about any changes in the skin, such as itching, warmth, redness, rashes, blisters, or growths. The incidence of skin cancer increases with age, and older adults should be asked specifically about skin growths that have changed in

size; are sore, open, cracked, itchy, or bleeding, or simply will not heal. Because older adults may also have visual changes, which makes early visual recognition of skin changes difficult, ask them if they have noted any new rough areas of their skin that do not seem to go away.

COGNITION AND AFFECTIVE STATES

Although traditionally considered within the neurological system, it is useful to consider common psychological problems associated with aging in a separate review of systems. The three important areas to focus on are cognitive status, mood, and sleep disorders. A review of the patient's cognitive status and current changes in cognition is essential to differentiate among dementia, depression, and delirium, which is potentially reversible. Obviously, when there are concerns about cognition, history taking will need to include the family and/or caregivers as well as the patient.

In the confused older adult, it is often difficult to determine whether the confusion is due to delirium, an underlying dementia, or depression. These conditions may occur independently or together. Table 3.11 highlights the differences among the three conditions. The confusion most commonly associated with dementia is gradual and irreversible and is associated with progressive memory loss. In contrast, delirium develops suddenly, is reversible, becomes worse at night, and is associated with inattentiveness and disturbances of thinking and perception. Depression, a disorder of

TABLE 3.11 Characteristics of Dementia, Delirium, and Depression

Feature	Dementia	Delirium	Depression
Onset	Gradual	Abrupt (hours to weeks)	Either
Prognosis	Irreversible	Reversible	Variable
Course	Progressive	Worse in p.m.	Worse in a.m.
Attention	Normal	Impaired	Variable
Memory	Impaired recent and remote	Impaired recent and immediate	Selective impairment
Perception	Normal	Impaired	Normal
Psychomotor behavior	Normal/ Apraxia	Hypo/ Hyperkinetic	Retardation/ Agitation

mood, has variable onset and duration, although generally the symptoms of depression are worse in the morning. History taking should focus on identifying the common causes of delirium in older adults, which include acute illness, infection, dehydration, electrolyte imbalance, medications, and environmental challenges.

Depression is the most common psychiatric disorder in older adults, but it is one of the most misdiagnosed, underdiagnosed, and undertreated illnesses experienced by older adults. Older adults may not recognize the signs and symptoms of depression, or they may be unwilling to report them to a health care provider because of the stigma involved. Table 3.12 reviews the typical and atypical signs and symptoms the patient may experience with depression. Explore when these symptoms were first noted, and any specific life events that may have occurred at the same time (a death in the family, loss of a friend or pet, or a move).

A variety of tools can be used in assessment of memory, mood, and the common behaviors associated with dementia, depression, and delirium (Table 3.13). These tools can help guide the clinician or caregiver on the signs and symptoms to look for to help identify changes, and they are particularly useful with cognitively impaired older adults who may not recognize that they have a physical problem, such as a pneumonia, but do demonstrate signs and symptoms of delirium.

Sleep changes and disorders are a common complaint for older adults and thus should be included in the history. Some of these changes may be due to the nor-

TABLE 3.13   Cognitive and Behavioral Measurement Tools

Focus of Assessment	Tools
Agitation	Cohen-Mansfield Agitation Index
Anxiety	HAM-A (Hamilton Anxiety Inventory)
	MSPS (Marks Sheehan Phobia Scale
Function	DAD (Disability Assessment for Dementia)
	PDS (Progressive Deterioration Scale)
	GDS I (Global Deterioration Scale)
	FAST (Functional Assessment Staging)
Depression	HAM-D (Hamilton Depression Inventory)
	GDS (Geriatric Depression Scale)
Obsessive-compulsive disorder	Y-BOCS (Yale-Brown Obsessive Compulsive Scale)
Psychosis	PANSS (Positive and Negative Syndrome Scale)
Behavior	BEHAVE-AD (Behavioral Pathology in AD Scale
	BPRS (Brief Psychiatric Rating Scale)

mal process of aging (Table 3.14), and others may be due to psychosocial issues that affect sleep. Explore with older adults when the sleep disorder began, its duration and severity, and how the change in sleep affects their life. Ask about difficulty falling asleep, difficulty staying asleep, feeling rested in the morning, snoring, and the existence of leg movement, pain, or jerking during the night that prevents them from falling asleep or wakes them during the night. Determine if the patient is having any associated symptoms that are influencing sleep, such as chest pain, indigestion, back pain, or urinary frequency. A review of sleep hygiene, caffeine use, and exercise/activity should also be done as it relates to sleep behavior. Be sure also to ask about napping during the day, the approximate length those naps, and the amount of time the individual spends in bed not sleeping. Roomates, caregivers, spouses, or significant

TABLE 3.12   Typical and Atypical Signs and Symptoms of Depression

Atypical Signs and Symptoms	Typical Signs and Symptoms
Vague somatic complaints, such as constipation, joint pain, fatigue, and memory changes	Changes in appetite
	Changes in sleep patterns
	Social withdrawal
The somatic complaints seem to be out of proportion to the actual problem, i.e., the patient is obsessed with the problems and feels that if they can be relieved he or she will be fine.	Loss of motivation
	Constipation
	Pessimism
	Guilt
	Decreased self-esteem
	Feelings of helplessness
	Hostility
	Agitation
	Aggression
	Anxiety

TABLE 3.14   Age-Related Changes in Sleep and the Sleep Cycle

- Longer time to fall asleep
- Increased time in Stage 1 and 2 sleep
- Decreased time in deeper stages of sleep (Stages 3 and 4)
- Decreased rapid eye movement (REM) sleep
- Increased and shorter repetition of the sleep cycle
- Increased night-time awakenings
- Altered circadian rhythm with a need to fall asleep earlier and awake earlier

others should also be asked about snoring or changes in breathing patterns and excessive leg movement or jerking during the night.

A careful assessment of cognition, mood, and sleep disorders is critical to identifying potentially reversible causes of disability and can greatly enhance the effectiveness of restorative care interventions.

PHYSICAL EXAM

The physical exam of older adults begins as soon as they enter the office or exam room, or the health care provider enters into their room. Observe the functional mobility of the patient, his or her overall appearance, particularly hygiene, and his or her ability to transfer from a chair to the exam table and to manage clothes. Vital signs should be obtained, including height and weight in a standardized fashion. If the scale being used requires a step up, be sure the patient is assisted for safety. In light of the increased risk and incidence of hypothermia in older adults, have available a reliable low-reading thermometer. To determine if there is evidence of orthostatic hypotension, blood pressures should be taken in the supine position after at least 10 minutes of rest, then immediately upon standing, and again 3 minutes after standing. Evaluate the heart rate response to postural changes at the same time because this provides important information about the cause of orthostatic hypotension. A rise of less than 10 beats per minute with a drop in blood pressure suggests baroreceptor reflex impairment.

Head

A common finding in the observation of the head in older adults is the presence of arcus senilis, or arcus ocularis or cornealis, or xanthelasma. This has no clinical significance, but is simply a descriptive finding. In light of the increased incidence of temporal arteritis in older adults, palpate the temporal arteries for pain, nodularity, and the presence of a pulse.

Testing of sensory function during the eye exam of older adults is essential. Visual acuity can be tested using a pocket Snellen chart held 14 inches from the eye. The patient can also be asked to read normal sized and/or enlarged print. Evaluation of extraocular movements and cranial nerves should be included. Fundo-

scopic examination in older adults may be difficult due to lens opacification and pupillary constriction. The exam, however, can provide important clues to the presence of systemic illness, glaucoma (increased cupping), or senile macular degeneration.

Hearing screening is imperative because of the large percentage of older adults with hearing impairment. The whispered voice test is a sensitive measure of hearing and can be easily followed over time (Lichtenstein, Bess, & Logan, 1988). If available, a handheld audioscope can also be used to test hearing. A referral to an audiologist should be made if the individual is unable to hear the 40dBHL tone in either ear (Weinstein, 1994). All older adults must have their ears evaluated for the buildup of cerumen, which can decrease hearing acuity by 40 to 45 dB. Removal of the cerumen corrects the impairment (Meador, 1995). In addition to looking for impacted cerumen, evaluate the external canal carefully for external otitis. Some older adults who wear hearing aids develop contact dermatitis in response to their hearing aids.

Evaluation of the neck should include range of movement, with consideration for evidence of dizziness while the patient is going through these position changes.

Cardiovascular System

The focus and interpretation of the cardiovascular exam in older adults differentiate this exam from a cardiac exam done in younger individuals. The jugular venous pulse should be palpated and the carotid arteries checked for bruits. It is challenging to differentiate a carotid bruit from a murmur that has radiated to the neck. In older adults, both atrial and ventricular ectopy are common, as is the evidence of S_4. However, the presence of an S_3 is indicative of congestive heart failure. Systolic ejection murmurs commonly occur and generally are due to hemodynamically insignificant aortic valve sclerosis. These are usually short, early-peaking murmurs that do not radiate to the neck and are graded II/VI. Conversely, aortic stenosis murmurs are generally louder, later-peaking, radiate to the neck, and are associated with a thrill and graded at a III/VI. Moreover, in patients with aortic stenosis there will be a diminution of the aortic component of S_2, a narrowed pulse pressure, and dampening of the carotid upstroke. Diastolic murmurs in older adults are always abnormal.

The most important aspect of the cardiac assessment of older adults in an evaluation for restorative care is to determine if the heart rate is within a normal limit and if it is regular. There is a high incidence of atrial fibrillation in this population, best heard as an irregularly irregular rhythm. If the rate is greater than 120 beats per minute, the individual may become dizzy due to poor perfusion. This rapid and irregular rate should be addressed so that the individual can function at his or her optimal physical level.

Peripheral vascular disease is very common in older adults. It is not unusual for there to be an absent dorsalis pedis or posterior tibial pulse. However, if both of these pulses are absent, further evaluation of the extremity for ischemia should be done. The classic signs of arterial insufficiency include pulselessness, pallor, pain, paresthesias, and paralysis. Laterally placed ulcers, cold and painful feet, gangrene, dependent rubor, and poor circulation in the toes are all indicative of arterial insufficiency. If a Doppler is available to determine pressures, a ratio of ankle pressure to brachial artery systolic pressure should be calculated. A ratio of <.80 confirms arterial insufficiency.

The lower extremities should also be evaluated for venous insufficiency. Evidence of pitting edema, medially and irregularly shaped ulcers with exudate, brawny skin discoloration, and stasis dermatitis are all indicative of venous insufficiency.

Respiratory System

Because of normal age changes and loss of elasticity of the chest wall, chest expansion may be decreased in older adults. It is not unusual for there to be basilar rales in the absence of disease. This is particularly true if the patient has evidence of kyphosis. These marginal or atelectatic crackles should disappear after the patient takes a few deep breaths.

Cough is another important clinical sign in older adults and may be related to congestive heart failure, pneumonia, an upper respiratory infection, or a malignancy. Observation of the cough, whether or not it is productive, and what the individual expectorates are useful to evaluate for diagnostic purposes and to help determine the need for further tests.

Endurance is a major problem for older adults with respiratory problems, such as chronic obstructive lung disease, and oxygen levels should be evaluated both at rest and during activity to determine if the individual is desaturating. A particularly important intervention is the use of oxygen if needed during times of activity. Use of oxygen will help the individual not only to achieve his or her highest functional level, but to do so more comfortably. If the oxygen level drops below 90% using pulse oximetry, then oxygen may be needed. If the individual appears to be short of breath but the oxygen saturation is within a normal range, it is possible that he or she is simply deconditioned. In this case, the individual should be encouraged to rest and then resume activity. This will help to increase endurance over time.

Gastrointestinal System

Begin the abdominal examination of the older adult with inspection. It is particularly important to recognize distention, the evidence of old scars (which may provide information about surgeries the individual forgot to mention in the history), and abdominal skin folds that may occur from osteoporosis and vertebral compression. Percussion of the abdomin in an older patient should include the bladder, in light of the increased incidence of urinary retention in both females and males of this age group. Percussion may also result in dullness over distal areas of the colon due to stool. A follow-up physical exam in these cases should be done to determine whether the dullness was in fact due to stool rather than a tumor.

Tortuosity or aneurysm of the abdominal aorta may be felt as a pulsatile mass in the abdomen. An aneurysm may have lateral as well as anteroposterior pulsation. Aneurysms are usually wider than 3 cm and often have an associated bruit. Surgical evaluation may be appropriate, particularly if the size of the aneurysm is greater than 5 cm and the individual is willing to pursue this option. Currently there are less invasive procedures (laproscopic surgery) to repair aneurysms, which should be considered if fear of rupture impedes the older individual's willingness to engage in functional activities.

Genitourinary System

Unless evidence of a genitourinary problem is identified in the history, an internal pelvic exam is generally not indicated for restorative care services. If evidence is discovered of a urinary disorder, a postvoid residual or bedside cystometry may be ordered to help determine the underlying cause of the incontinence, as previously described. One of the best interventions to improve urinary function, however, is to improve functional performance and thereby facilitate the older individual's ability to get to the bathroom in a timely fashion.

Musculoskeletal System

As previously indicated, the evaluation of this system is central to the development of a restorative care plan. Observe all joints for enlargement and inflammation. Heberden's nodes, involving the distal interphalangeal joints, are common but rarely inflamed. All joints in the older adult should be evaluated and range of motion tested. Ask the individual to actively range the joint, and only put the joint through passive range of motion if he or she is unable to do so independently. Table 3.15 provides a useful guide to evaluate all important joints related to restorative care activities. It is essential to actually observe what the individual's underlying capability is with regard to range because this relates to what the individual can do functionally. For example, if the individual has full range of motion in the hands, elbows, and shoulders, then he or she has the ability to self-feed. If there are cognitive problems, then cueing may be necessary. Conversely, if the individual has fixed flexion in both hands (all fingers), and the elbows are fixed in the flexed position, then he or she may not be able to self-feed, at least without the use of extensive adaptive equipment.

A number of functional tests can be used to evaluate the patient's functional performance. For upper extremity function, it is useful to ask the patient to touch the back of the head with hands (range of motion), pick up a penny (fine motor movement), and shake hands (grip strength) (Lachs, Feinstein & Cooney, 1990). To evaluate lower extremity function, the timed Get Up and Go measure can be used (Tinetti & Ginter, 1988). To do this test, ask the individual to rise from a standard chair without arms, walk 3 meters, turn, walk back, and sit down. Note the time it takes the individual to do the task. This is a particularly useful measure to follow the patient's mobility function over time.

Special attention should also be given to the feet of older adults. Diabetic-related ulcerations, fungal infec-

tions of the feet or toenails, calluses, bunions, hallus vagus (which is a lateral deviation of the large toe), and other deformities are very common and can affect function. Evaluate the footwear of the older adult, since improper footwear can cause pain, ulcerations, and falls.

Neurological System

With age come numerous commonly occurring changes in the neurological system that are not related to disease. Gait changes are a good example. Approximately half of those over 65 years of age demonstrate decreased arm swing during gait, although only a small percentage of those with abnormal gaits had an associated specific disease (Odenheimer, Funkenstein, & Beckett, 1994). All older adults should have muscle strength, cranial nerves, sensation, and reflexes checked. With regard to restorative care activities, it is most important that muscle muscle strength testing be done in all major muscle groups using standard gradings found in Table 3.16. The steps for manual muscle strength testing are shown in Table 3.17, and Table 3.18 provides a observation tool to record these baseline measures. Gaining a sense of the individual's strength will likewise help determine underlying capabilities and give both the caregiver and the older adult an opportunity to see improvements after regular restorative care activities. Upper extremity muscle strength could be easily improved with daily weight lifting in the dining room while the older individual waits for meals to arrive. Weights can be left on the tables for this reason, and caregivers can initiate a weight lifting session as residents wait.

Gait speed declines .2% per year up to age 63, and this decline increases up to 1.6% per year after age 63 (Dobbs, Charlett, & Bowes, 1993). The other characteristics of gait that change with aging include a decline in step length, stride length, ankle range of motion; decreased vertical and increased horizontal head excursions; decreased spinal rotation, decreased arm swing, increased length of double support phase of walking, and a reduction in propulsive force generalized at the push-off phase.

Older adults also have a decrease in sensory input, slowing of motor responses, and musculoskeletal limitations. The combination of these changes results in an increase in unsteadiness or postural sway under both static and dynamic conditions. Older adults compen-

TABLE 3.15   Contractures

When you measure contractures and muscle strength, the residents should be lying down. For most efficient use of your time, you may want to talk with the nursing assistants to determine the residents' schedules, for example what time the resident rises in the morning, whether the resident goes to bed after lunch.

Contractures should be evaluated by putting the joint through active or passive range of motion. Active range of motion should be tried first and if the resident is unable then passive range of motion used. Adequate space for the resident to move each muscle group and joint through its full range is necessary. Instruct the resident to move each joint through its range of motion as described below. If the resident does not complete full-range actively, put the joint through the remaining range, stopping at the point of pain. Use a goniometer to measure the angle. Begin with the joint in the fully extended or neutral position and then flex the joint as far as possible. Measure the angles of greatest flexion and extension by placing circle over joint. Compare normal expected ranges with results of goniometer assessment to determine evidence of contracture. Normal ranges are listed below.

DESCRIPTION OF NORMAL RANGES:

Hand
Hand closes in a tight fist, and hand opens to a flat surface

Wrist
Flexion: 80–90 degrees   Bend wrist so palm nears lower arm
Extension: 70 degrees   Bend wrist in opposite direction
Radial deviation: 20 degrees   Bend wrist so thumb nears radius
Ulnar deviation: 30–50   Bend wrist so pinky finger nears ulna
   degrees

Elbow
Flexion: 150 degrees   Bring lower arm to the biceps
Extension: 180 degrees   Straighten out lower arm
Supination: 90 degrees   Turn lower arm so palm of hand
                                     faces up
Pronation: 90 degrees   Turn lower arm so palm faces down

Shoulder
Abduction: 180 degrees   Bring arm up sideways
Adduction: 45 degrees   Bring arm toward the midline of
                                     the body
Horizontal extension: Swing arm horizontally backward
   45 degrees
Horizontal flexion: 130 degrees Swing arm horizontally forward
Vertical extension: 60 degrees Raise arm straight backward
Vertical flexion: 180 degrees   Raise arm straight forward

Ankle
Flexion: 45 degrees   Bend ankle so toes point up
Extension: 20 degrees   Bend ankle so toes point down
Pronation: 30 degrees   Turn foot so the sole faces in
Supination: 20 degrees   Turn foot so the sole faces out.

Knee
Flexion: 130 degrees   Touch calf to hamstring.
Extension: 15 degrees   Straighten out knee as much as
                                     possible
Internal rotation: 10 degrees   Twist lower leg toward midline

Hip
Flexion: 110–130 degrees   Flex knee and bring thigh close to
                                     abdomen
Extension: 30 degrees   Move thigh backward without
                                     moving the pelvis
Abduction: 45–50 degrees   Swing thigh away from midline
Adduction: 20–30 degrees   Bring thigh toward and across
                                     midline
Internal rotation: 40 degrees   Flex knee and swing lower leg
                                     away from midline
External rotation: 45 degrees   Flex knee and swing lower leg
                                     toward midline

Introduction to Patients: I'd like to see how you move your hands, shoulders, and legs. I would like you to try to imitate what I do. Then I may try to move your arms or legs for you. If it is painful, please tell me immediately.

Circle Yes if there is evidence for a contracture as compared to standards above.

	Yes = 1	No = 2
1. Right Hand	1	2
2. Left Hand	1	2
3. Right Wrist	1	2
4. Left Wrist	1	2
5. Right Elbow	1	2
6. Left Elbow	1	2
7. Right Shoulder	1	2
8. Left Shoulder	1	2
9. Right Ankle	1	2
10. Left Ankle	1	2
11. Right Knee	1	2
12. Left Knee	1	2
13. Right Hip	1	2
14. Left Hip	1	2

TABLE 3.16　Muscle Strength Grading

Grade	Definition
0	Flaccid
1	Trace/slight contractility but no movement
2	Weak, but movement possible when gravity is eliminated
3	Fair movement against gravity but not against resistance
4	Good with movement against gravity with some resistance
5	Normal with movement against gravity and some resistance

sate for changes by using sensory input to augment proprioceptive loss. Observe the gait of the older adult, taking note of the steppage height, ability to walk on uneven surfaces, transfer ability, and any unsteadiness during walking. Common gait disorders in older adults are described in Table 3.19. Also evaluate balance, both sitting and standing. Standing balance can be tested using the Romberg and/or a sternal nudge to determine if the individual can respond to this challenge. Observing the older adult perform the Get Up and Go test also provides useful information about balance.

Cognition and Affective States

Cognitive screening to establish baseline ability is essential when working with older adults. The Mini-Mental State Examination (MMSE) (Folstein, Fol-

TABLE 3.17　Steps for Doing Manual Muscle Testing

Instructions to Participant: Now I would like to test your muscle strength. I will ask you to perform a few exercises that measure your muscle strength. For each movement, I will first describe and show the movement to you. Then I'd like you to do it. If you cannot do a particular movement or you feel it would be unsafe to try to do it, tell me and we'll move on to the next one. Let me emphasize that I do not want you to do any exercise you feel might be unsafe. To test your muscles, all you have to do is push against me.

Upper Extremity

1. *Shoulder extension:* Have the resident hold up his/her arm at 90 degrees. Place your hand on the resident's upper arm between elbow and shoulder and tell the resident not to let you push down his/her arm.
2. *Elbow flexion:* Have the resident bend his/her elbow fully and attempt to straighten the arm out while telling the resident not to let you pull the arm down.
3. *Elbow extension:* While the resident still has the elbow flexed, tell him/her to try to straighten out the arm while you resist.

Lower Extremity:

1. *Hip flexion:* Place your hand on the resident's anterior thigh and ask him/her to raise the leg against your resisting hand. (Say to resident, "Don't let me push your leg down.")
2. *Knee extension:* Have the resident bend his/her leg on the bed. Place one of your hands just below the resident's knee and tell him/her to try to straighten out the leg as you resist.
3. *Ankle plantar flexion:* Have the resident extend his/her foot against your hand.
4. *Ankle dorsiflexion:* Have the resident pull his or her foot up against your hand.

TABLE 3.18　Tool to Record Muscle Strength

	Flaccid 0	Trace 1	Weak 2	Fair 3	Good 4	Normal 5
1. Right shoulder extension	0	1	2	3	4	5
2. Left shoulder extension	0	1	2	3	4	5
3. Right elbow extension	0	1	2	3	4	5
4. Left elbow extension	0	1	2	3	4	5
5. Right elbow flexion	0	1	2	3	4	5
6. Left elbow flexion	0	1	2	3	4	5
7. Right ankle extension (plantar flexion)	0	1	2	3	4	5
8. Left ankle extension (plantar flexion)	0	1	2	3	4	5
9. Right ankle flexion (dorsiflexion)	0	1	2	3	4	5
10. Left ankle flexion (dorsiflexion)	0	1	2	3	4	5
11. Right knee extension	0	1	2	3	4	5
12. Left knee extension	0	1	2	3	4	5
13. Right hip flexion	0	1	2	3	4	5
14. Left hip flexion	0	1	2	3	4	5

TABLE 3.19   Gait Disorders

Type of Gait	Description of Gait	Type of Gait	Description of Gait
Frontal lobe gait	Wide base of support Slightly flexed posture Small, shuffling, hesitant steps Poor initiation of gait; "slipping clutch syndrome" Turns by pivoting both feet in a small circle Can't control changes in base of support	Antalgic and gonalgic gait (cont.)	Decreased stance and swing phases of gait Decreased walking velocity Knee and foot flexed Decreased hip and knee extension Limp due to leg length discrepancies
		Podalgic gait	Pain with ambulation Toe contact occurs for 3/4 of the gait cycle
Sensory ataxic gait	Wide-based stance; "foot stamping walk" High step/stamping walk Heel touches first then foot stamps Visual input used to ambulate + Romberg sign	Dementia-related gait	Decreased walking speed Decreased step length Increased double support time Increase step-to-step variability Increased postural sway Flexed posture Apraxic gait
Cerebellar ataxic gait	Wide-based stance Small, irregular, unsteady steps Drunken veering and lurching Impaired trunk control Difficulty with tandem gait Turns en bloc	Festinating gait	Symmetric rapid shuffling of feet Trunk bent forward, hips and knees flexed Difficulty stepping
Spastic gait	Swings affected leg slowly in outward arc; circumduction of the leg Legs trace a semicircle when walking Feet scrape the ground Scissoring occurs Short steps Narrow base	Parkinsonian gait	Festination Marche a petits pas; short, flat-footed shuffles Delayed gait initiation Body moves forward before feet Freezing Wide stance En bloc turning Loss of postural control
Spastic paraparesis	Legs move slowly in a stiff manner Short, labored steps with decreased hip and knee movement (bilateral circumduction) Toes scrape the ground Scissoring occurs Short steps Narrow base		Retropulsion; falls back in one piece like a log Propulsion
		Waddling gait	Lateral trunk movement away from the foot with exaggerated rotation of the pelvis and rolling of hips Difficulty with stairs and chair rise
Steppage gait	Feet lifted high off the ground to prevent scraping toes Toes hit first, then heels Head down to observe foot placement	Vestibular ataxic gait	Broad based with frequent side stepping Drift toward the side of vestibular impairment Unsteady
Peripheral vestibular imbalance	Unsteady gait	Cautious gait	Flexed posture Decreased stride length Decreased walking speed Low center of gravity Wide based Short steps Turning en bloc
Antalgic and gonalgic gait	Reluctant to put weight on the joint Heel strike avoided on affected foot Push off avoided		

stein, & McHugh, 1975) is an easy bedside screening tool to evaluate cognitive function. It is adjusted for the educational level, and the individual's behavior during testing is a useful indicator of whether he or she has dementia, delirium, or depression. Individuals with dementia will work hard to answer the questions, and will confabulate answers. Those with delirium will have difficulty concentrating on the questions and attending to the task. Individuals with depression often are unwilling to try to complete the task or answer the questions. Alternatively, to test cognitive function, give the older adult a circle and ask him or her to draw a clock (Watson, Arfken, & Birge, 1993). This test is believed to be more sensitive to executive control

(Royall, Mulroy, Chiodo, & Polk, 1999). Scoring of the clock is described in Table 3.20.

In addition to cognition, mood is also important to evaluate in older adults. This evaluation includes observation of the individuals behavior in the office, his or her affect, and willingness to engage in the examination and looking for evidence of the typical and atypical signs and symptoms of depression, but several screening tools can also be used. As previously indicated, there are numerous measures for depression in older adults, but it is often easiest clinically to simply use the Single Item Yale Depression Screening Tool and ask older patient, "Do you often feel sad or depressed?" (Mahoney et al., 1994). This was shown to correlate very closely with the 15-item Geriatric Depression Scale (GDS) (Resnick, 1998).

Integumentary System

Older adults commonly present with dry, scaly skin; hyperpigmented macular lesions referred to as lentigines or "liver" spots; and seborrheic keratoses, which are benign pigmented lesions with a waxy surface, on the face and trunk. Skin turgor is normally decreased in older adults and should not be used as a marker of hydration status. Senile purpura, commonly found on the hands and forearms, is due to the frail nature of capillaries and decreased collagen support. Actinic keratoses commonly occur in older adults on sun-exposed areas of the skin. These are premalignant lesions and can grow, but they usually grow relatively slowly.

Skin folds—particularly folds in the abdomin, under breasts, in the groin, and between toes—should be aggressively evaluated for fungal infections. Older women who are kyphotic may develop fungal rashes in abdominal crevices because of constant skin-on-skin exposure and poor hygiene in these areas.

Malignant skin lesions, particularly, basal cell and squamous cell carcinomas, are also common in older adults. Generally these growths are found on sun-exposed areas, although they also can occur on extremities or even on the trunk. Basal cell carcinomas tend to be pearly, papular, or plaquelike lesions that may be ulcerated in the center. They may present as lesions that simply do not heal. Squamous cell carcinomas tend to be erythematous, indurated areas that may be scaly or hyperkeratotic. These tend to grow more rapidly than basal cell carcinomas. Melanomas, in contrast, are pigmented macular or nodular lesions with irregular borders.

All skin should be examined for areas of pressure and/or pressure sores. Ecchymoses should also be noted, and if they are identified, an attempt should be made to determine if there was a traumatic cause.

SITE-SPECIFIC EVALUATION TOOLS

Depending on the site of care, other assessment tools may be required. Components of these can be used to help consider underlying function and build restorative care activities to augment baseline function. In long-term care sites, the Minimum Data Set (MDS) is required (http://cms.hhs.gov/medicaid/mds20/default.asp). The MDS has several sections relevant to restorative care that provide at least a basic assessment of the individual's current function, behavior, and cognitive status. Similarly, in the home setting the Outcome and Assessment Information Set (OASIS) must be completed on all patients receiving home care serv-

TABLE 3.20 Clock Drawing Scoring

Option One

1. Divide the circle into 4 quadrants by drawing perpendicular lines through the center of the circle.
2. Count the number of digits in each quadrant in the clockwise direction beginning at the digit corresponding to number 12. Each digit is counted only once. If a digit falls on one of the reference lines, it is included in the quadrant that is clockwise to the line. Any three digits in a quadrant is considered to be correct.
3. For any error in the number of digits in the first, second, or third quadrants, assign a score of 1. For any error in the number of digits in the fourth quadrant assign a score of 4.
4. Normal range of score is 0 to 3. Abnormal score is 4 and above.

Option II

1. Evaluate only the fourth quadrant.
2. There should be three digits in this quadrant. If a digit falls on one of the reference lines, it is included in the quadrant that is clockwise to the line.
3. Scoring is as follows:
   0=3 numbers were correct in the quadrant.
   1=2 numbers were correct in the quadrant.
   2=1 number was correct in the quadrant.
   3=0 numbers were correct in the quadrant.
   4=more than 3 numbers were in the quadrant.

ices. Like the MDS, this assessment tool guides the clinician to do a very comprehensive review of the older adult, incorporating some general functional assessments (http://cms.hhs.gov/oasis/all.pdf). In the assisted living setting, the required assessment varies state by state. Maryland, for example, provides a comprehensive tool that includes an assessment of the ability to perform not only activities of daily living, but also instrumental activities of daily living such as taking medications and preparing meals. In many states, however, no specific assessment is required. In those states, facilities would benefit by incorporating any of the tools recommended in this chapter to help evaluate underlying functional abilities and to guide caregivers in developing a restorative care program.

SCREENING FOR EXERCISE ACTIVITIES

All types of physical activity (Table 3.21) when done regularly, have important health benefits, and encouraging individuals to exercise is an important goal of

TABLE 3.21   Exercise Definitions

Physical activity: bodily movement produced by skeletal muscles that requires energy expenditure and produces progressive health benefits.

Exercise: a type of physical activity defined as a planned, structured, and repetitive bodily movement done to improve or maintain one or more components of physical fitness.

Aerobic exercise: Physical activity that stimulates mitochondrial oxidative metabolism. It is typified by repetitive large muscle group movement that does not result in progressive blood stream lactic acid accumulation (e.g., walking, cycling, running).

Resistive exercise: Training with resistance to movement to increase muscle strength through the use of weights, bands, air pressure, or one's own body weight (e.g., pushups).

Isometric exercise: Exertion during which the muscle does not change length (e.g., pushing an immovable object).

Moderate activity: Activity that results in the individual maintaining a heart rate that is 60–80% of his or her targeted heart rate. Examples include:

Washing windows/floors for 45–60 minutes
Gardening for 40 minutes
Wheeling self in wheelchair for 40 minutes
Walking 1¾ mile in 35 minutes
Bicycling 4 miles in 15 minutes
Running 1¾ miles in 15 minutes
Stairwalking for 15 minutes

health care. The question remains, however, of how much exercise is needed to achieve these health benefits. The National Institutes of Health Consensus Development Conference (1995) "Physical Activity and Cardiovascular Health" concluded that the majority of benefits of physical activity can be gained by performing moderate-intensity activity outside of exercise.

To optimize safety during exercise participation and to permit the development of a sound and effective exercise program, participants must have an initial screening relative to important health factors. The degree of screening can range from self-administered questionnaires to expensive and sophisticated diagnostic tests. Older adults, that is, adults 70 years of age and above, who have not previously been active check with their health care provider prior to starting an exercise program. For these individuals, the extent of prescreening needed prior to starting an exercise program relates to the individual's current health status. The American College of Sports Medicine (1995) recommends that individuals be categorized as follows: (1) Low risk individuals are healthy with no more than one of the risk factors for coronary heart disease (high blood cholesterol, high blood pressure, diabetes, cigarette smoking, obesity, or a sedentary lifestyle). (2) Higher risk individuals have two or more of the risk factors for coronary heart disease. This category is further broken down into those with symptoms (i.e., chest pain or shortness of breath) and those without symptoms. (3) Individuals with chronic disease such as heart, lung, or metabolic disease. Once the individual is categorized, a decision can be made about whether a complete medical evaluation or stress testing is needed prior to starting an exercise program (Table 3.22). Interestingly,

TABLE 3.22   Need for Prescreening of Older Adults for Safe Exercise

Type of Activity	Low Risk, Healthy Individual	High Risk, No Symptoms	High Risk, Symptoms	Chronic Disease
Low intensity < 60% MHR*	No	No	No	No
Moderate intensity < 60–80% MHR	No	No	Yes	Yes
Vigorous activity > 80% MHR	Yes	Yes	Yes	Yes

*MHR is the individual's maximum heart rate, which is calculated as 220 minus age.

TABLE 3.23 Warning Signs to Recognize During Exercise

- Pale, clammy, cool skin
- Change in cognition—confusion or disorientation
- Nausea or vomiting
- Shortness of breath that does not resolve in 30 minutes
- Chest pain
- Dizziness
- Unusual fatigue
- A change in balance or unsteadiness

there are no specific screening tools for resistance exercise. Good common sense should be used, however, and older adults should be aware of pain in muscles and joints and avoid pushing beyond the pain during exercise sessions. Likewise, older adults and caregivers should be familiar with the warning signs to recognize during aerobic activity (Table 3.23).

PULLING IT ALL TOGETHER

Once the caregiver or caregiving team has had the opportunity to do a comprehensive evaluation of the older individual, the information obtained should be used to develop the plan of care, as described in chapter 4. It is often hard to rationalize taking the time to assess older individuals when care providers need the time to provide services. It is essential, however, to take this time and carefully evaluate underlying function and abilities from gait patterns, range of motion, sensation, and hearing. Knowing what resources are available within the individual is the first step to helping him or her obtain optimal function. Care providers have the responsibility to build off these resources, encourage optimal function, and motivate the older adult to use his or her capabilities to perform functional activities, to exercise, and ideally to achieve his or her highest level of health and function. Subsequent chapters focus on the many ways in which care providers can build off the basic assessment in order to engage older individuals in restorative care activities.

REFERENCES

American College of Sports Medicine Recommendations for cardiovascular screening, staffing, and emergency policies at health fitness facilities. Medicine Science, Sports & Exercise (1998), 25(4), 1009–1078.

Daly, M., & Adelman, A. (2000). Nutritional Status and Involuntary Weight Loss. In: Adelman, A. & Daly, M. 20 Common Problems in Geriatrics, New York: McGraw-Hill.

Dobbs, R., Charlett, A., & Bowes, S. (1993). Is this walk normal? *Age and Ageing, 22,* 27–30.

Folstein, M., Folstein, S., & McHugh, P. (1975). Mini-mental state: A practical method for grading the cognitive state of patients for the clinician. *Journal of Psychiatric Research, 12,* 189–198.

Fries, J.F., Spitz, P.W., & Young, D.Y. (1982). The dimensions of health outcomes: The health assessment questionnaire, disability and pain scales. *Journal of Rheumatology, 9,* 789–793.

Hamilton, B.B., Granger, C.V., Sherwin, F.S., et al. (1987). A uniform national data system for Rehabilitation outcomes: analysis and measurement. Baltimore, MD: Paul H. Brookes, 137–147.

Jette, A.M. (1982). Functional capacity evaluation: An empirical approach. *Archives of Physical Medicine and Rehabilitation, 61,* 85–89.

Jette, A.M., & Deniston, O.L. (1978). Inter-observer reliability of a functional status assessment instrument. *Journal of Chronic Disease, 31,* 573–580.

Kaasa, T., Loomis, J., Gillis, K., et al. (1997). The Edmonton functional assessment tool: Preliminary development and evaluation for use in palliative care. *Journal of Pain Symptom Management, 13,* 10–19.

Katz, S., Ford, A., & Moskowitz, R. (1963) Studies of illness in the aged: The index of ADL. *Journal of the American Medical Association, 185,* 914–919.

Lachs, M., Feinstein, A., & Cooney, L. (1990). A simple procedure for general screening of functional disability in elderly patients. *Annals of Internal Medicine, 112,* 699–702.

Lawton, M.P., & Brody, E. (1969). Assessment of older people: Self-maintaining and instrumental activities of daily living. *Gerontologist, 9,* 179–186.

Lichtenstein, M., Bess, F., & Logan, S. (1988). Validation of screening tools for identifying hearing-impaired elderly in primary care. *Journal of the American Medical Association, 259,* 2875–2878.

Linn, M.W., & Linn, B.S. (1982). The rapid disability rating scale—2. *Journal of the American Geriatrics Society, 30,* 378–382.

Mahoney, F., & Barthel, D. (1965). Functional evaluation: The Barthel index. *Maryland State Medical Journal, 14*(2), 61–65.

Mahoney, J., Drinka, T., Abler, R., Gunter-Hunt, G., Matthews, C., Gravenstein, S., & Carnes, M. (1994). Screening for depression: Single question versus

GDS. *Journal of the American Geriatrics Society, 42,* 1006–1007.

Mariotto, A., Warren, J. L., Knopf, K. B., Feurer, B. J. (2003). The prevalence of patients with colorectal carcinoma under care in the U.S. *Cancer, 91*(6), 1253–1261.

Meador, J. (1995). Cerumen impaction in the elderly. *Journal of Gerontological Nursing, 25,* 43–45.

Nelson, E.C., Wasson, J.H., Johnson, D.J., & Hays, R.D. (1996). Dartmouth COOP functional health assessment charts: Brief measures for clinical practice. In B. Spilker (Ed.), *Quality of life in pharmacoeconomics in clinical trials.* Philadelphia: Lippincott-Raven Publishers. p. 137–148.

Nesher, G., & Moore, T. (1994). Clinical presentation and treatment of arthritis in the elderly. *Clinics in Geriatric Medicine, 10,* 659–675.

Odenheimer, G., Funkenstein, H., & Beckett, L. (1994). Comparison of neurologic changes in "successfully aging" persons vs the total aging population. *Archives of Neurology, 51,* 573–580.

Parker, J., Vukov, L., & Wollan, P. (1996). Abdominal pain in the elderly: Use of temperature and laboratory testing to screen for surgical disease. *Family Medicine 28,* 193–197.

Patrick, D.L., Darby, S.C., Green, S., et al. (1981). Screening for disability in the inner city. *Journal of Epidemiology and Community Health, 35,* 65–70.

Pfeffer, R.I., Kurosaki, T.T., Chance, J.M. et al. (1984). Use of the Mental Function Index in older adults: Reliability, validity, and measurement of change over time. *American Journal of Epidemiology, 120,* 922–935.

Resnick, B. (1998). Functional performance of older adults in a long term care setting. Clinical Nursing Research, 7, 230–246.

Resnick, B. (1999). Atrial fibrillation in the older adult: Presentation and management. *Geriatric Nursing, 20,* 1–6.

Royall, D., Mulroy, A., Chiodo, L., & Polk, M. (1999). Clock drawing is sensitive to executive control: A comparison of six methods. *Journal of Gerontology, 54B,* P328–P333.

Sallis, J.F., Husluell, W.L., Wood, P.D., Furtmann, S.P., Rogers, T., Blair, S.N., Pafferberger, R.J. Jr. (1985). Physical activity assessment methodology in the five-city projects. *American Journal of Epidemiology, 121*(1), 91–106.

Schoening, H.A., Anderegg, L., Bergstrom, D., et al. (1965). Numerical scoring of self-care status of patients. *Archives of Physical Medicine and Rehabilitation, 46,* 689–697.

Schoening, H.A., & Iversen, I.A. (1968). Numerical scoring of self-care status: A study of the Kenny self-care evaluation. *Archives of Physical Medicine and Rehabilitation, 49,* 221–229.

Stewart, A., & Kamberg, C.J. (1992). Physical functioning measures. In A. Stewart & J.E. Ware (Eds.). *Measuring functioning and well-being: The medical outcomes study approach* (pp. 86–101). Durham, North Carolina: Duke University Press.

Tinetti, M., & Ginter, S. (1988). Identifying mobility dysfunctions in elderly patients: Standard neuormuscular examination or direct assessment? *Journal of the American Medical Association, 259,* 1190–1193.

Watson, Y., Arfken, C., & Birge, S. (1993). Clock completion: An objective screening test for dementia. *Journal of the American Geriatrics Society, 41,* 1235–1240.

Weinstein, B. (1994). Age related hearing loss: How to screen for it and when to intervene. *Geriatrics, 49,* 40–46.

CHAPTER 4

Restorative Care Activities

Robin E. Remsburg

Restorative care includes nursing interventions that assist or promote older adults' ability to attain their maximum functional potential. This does not include procedures or techniques carried out by or under the direction of a qualified therapist, but instead nursing interventions that promote older adults' ability to adapt and adjust to living as independently and safely as possible. Restorative care includes the following activities: walking and mobility exercises, dressing, grooming, eating, swallowing, transferring, amputation/prosthesis care, communication skills, and self-care skills such as diabetic management, ostomy care, or self-administration of medication.

THE RESTORATIVE CARE PROCESS

Capitalize on Remaining Abilities and Strengths

The restorative process can be viewed as a sequence of progressing actions ranging from minimal action by the caregiver to complete assistance when appropriate. The sequence capitalizes on the individual's remaining abilities and strengths, creates an enabling environment, breaks down tasks and provides the appropriate assistance, and includes repetition and practice to attain or maintain the individual's highest level of function (Remsburg, 1999b). As described in previous chapters, an important preliminary aspect of restorative care requires identification of the individual's limitations and strengths. Strategies and techniques to improve function should preserve residents' existing abilities and build on functional strengths.

Establishing appropriate achievable performance goals is essential in restorative care. For some older adults complete independence in self-care may be a realistic goal, but for others participation in some component part of self-care, such as combing hair or washing face, may be all that is reasonable to accomplish. Establishing a goal gives both the resident and the caregiver a target to work toward, and when it is achieved, both the resident and caregiver will experience a sense of accomplishment and satisfaction (Remsburg, Armacost, Radu, & Bennett, 1999). Measuring progress and outcomes of restorative care at regularly scheduled intervals not only documents the effectiveness of the care but also can motivate and encourage goal attainment. Table 4.1 provides examples of a Goal Attainment Scale that can be used to determine when a goal has actually been achieved.

Create an Enabling Environment

Another important aspect in restorative care activities is preparation and modification of the environment. For many older adults, rearranging the environment, for example, placing grooming dressing supplies within reach, removing barriers such as lids on coffee cups, or pouring milk from a carton into a cup, may facilitate self-care. For residents with cognitive impairment, removing noxious stimuli, such as noise from a television; enhancing the dining room atmosphere; or playing soothing music in the tub room can promote self-care activities.

Part of altering the environment to facilitate restorative care activities includes making appropriate tools for restorative care easily available to the older individual. Using assistive devices to augment self-

Table 4.1 Goal Attainment Scales

Level Of Predicted Attainment	Scale 1: Score	Scale 2: Bathing	Scale 3: Dressing	Eating
Much less than expected	(−2)	Bathed by staff	Dressed by staff	Fed by staff
Somewhat less than the expected level of outcome	(−1)	Lathers hair and underarms only	Only pulls on shirt and pants	Only grasps feeding utensils
Expected level of outcome	0	Bathes completely with directions from staff	Dresses completely with directions from staff	Feeds self with directions from staff
Somewhat more than the expected level of outcome	(+1)	Reminded to wash soap from underarms	Reminded only to put on socks	Needs reminders to finish meal
Much more than the expected level of outcome	(+2)	Bathes independently	Dresses independently	Eats independently

care deficits, such as buttoning devices or adaptive feeding utensils, promotes independence in self-care and be all that is necessary to achieve independence in self-care (Table 4.2). Many assistive devices, such as built-up eating utensils and walkers, require prescription by an occupational or physical therapist and an order from a physician. Device and equipment venders and occupational and physical therapists should be consulted for proper use of the prescribed devices or specialized equipment. A Merry Walker, for example, is an excellent way to augment ambulation in an older individual who may otherwise be at risk for falling when ambulating independently. Proper cleaning, storage, and maintenance should follow manufacturer guidelines.

Break Down Tasks and Provide the Appropriate Assistance

To facilitate performance of a restorative care activity, break the activity down into its component parts, such as holding the spoon, scooping the food, lifting the loaded spoon to the mouth. Component parts of activities of daily living (ADLs) are displayed in Table 4.3. For older adults with cognitive impairment, appropriate assistance from caregivers (e.g., cueing or prompting to eat or begin dressing) may be all that is required to preserve self-care performance. The skillful restorative caregiver is able to break the ADL activity down to its component parts, encourage the older adult to do the part of the activity that he/she can accomplish in-

Table 4.2 Assistive Devices for ADLs

Eating	Bathing	Grooming	Dressing	Toileting	Mobility	Exercise
Specialty utensils	Towels	Long-handled combs, brushes	Reachers	Bedside commode	*Positioning*	Weights
Built up spoon, fork, knife	Plastic bags	Nail brush & suction cups	Built on fastener	Raised toilet seat	Elbow & heel protectors	Elastic exercise bands
Bracelet handled spoon, fork	Soap on a rope	Builtup toothbrush	Stocking aid	Grab bars	Foot supports	Resistive exercise equipment
Weighted spoon, fork, knife	Soap dispenser	Builtup razor	Long-handled shoe horn	Fracture bed pan	Hand cones	Inflated balls
Two-handled cups	Wet wipes	Electric razor	Step stools	Urinals	Lap boards	Scarves
Sip cups	Water cleaners	Electric toothbrush	Zipper pulls	Toileting handles	Pillows	Sponge balls
Long straws	Long-handled sponges	Water pick	Oversize clothes	Waterfree cleansers	Seat cushions	Bicycle peddles
Plateguards	Wash mitten		Modified clothes & Velcro		Side rails	
Partitioned plates	Tub chair				Splints	
Rimmed plates					Trochanter rolls	
No slip mats					Wedges	
Mechanical feeders					*Transfers*	

Table 4.3 Components of ADLs

Eating	Bathing	Grooming	Dressing	Toileting	Mobility
Open milk cartons, straws, butter, sugar, and salt	Obtain bathing supplies	Pick up comb and brush	Obtain clothing	Inform staff of need to void	Moves head, neck, shoulders, arms, waist, hips, legs, feet
Hold fork, spoon, knife	Wet and apply soap to washcloth	Comb or brush hair	Put on and take off underpants	Inform staff of need to have a bowel movement	Lifts upper torso
Cut meat	Wring out washcloth	Pick up toothbrush	Put on and take off bra	Walk or wheel to the bathroom	Rolls from side to side
Butter bread	Wash and dry hands	Put toothpaste on brush	Put on and take off shirt	Transfer to the toilet or bedside commode	Lifts hips
Scoop food with spoon	Wash and dry face	Brush teeth or dentures	Put on and take off pants	Remove and replace undergarments	Grasps side rails
Spear food with fork	Wash and dry arms	Put in and take out dentures	Put on and take off socks	Dry and clean perineum and rectum	Pushes/pulls upper body off bed/chair
Lift loaded utensil to mouth and take a bite	Wash and dry chest and abdomen	Apply shaving cream	Put on and take off shoes	Wash and dry hands	Sits
Hold cup or glass	Wash and dry legs	Pick up razor	Tie, buckle, or fasten shoes	Roll from side to side	Stands up
Lift cup or glass to mouth and drink	Wash and dry feet	Shave face	Button and unbutton clothing	Lift up buttocks using a trapeze bar or side rail	Weight bears
Sip from a straw	Wash and dry back	Soak fingernails in water basin	Pull zipper up and down		Maintains balance
Hold a dinner roll	Wash and dry pubic area	Use nailbrush	Put on and take off glasses		Takes steps
Bring dinner roll to mouth and take a bite	Wash and dry rectal area	Use nail file or clippers	Put on or take off hearing aid or amplifier		
		Open makeup containers			
		Apply makeup to face			

dependently, and augment or assist in the parts of the activity the individual is unable to perform. It is unlikely that all older adults will return to complete independence in ADLs. Over time, many will experience declining abilities as medical conditions worsen, periodic acute exacerbations of chronic conditions occur, or new conditions develop. Though declines in function occur, most older adults retain the ability to perform some parts of their activities of daily living.

In addition to breaking the ADL activity down into its component parts, the caregiver is encouraged to use the system of least prompts (SLP) (Engelman, Mathews, Altus (2002). This system uses a hierarchy of prompts, starting with prompts that are the least intrusive and gradually proceeding to more intrusive prompts. Using the least amount of assistance necessary, individuals are able to complete ADLs.

Repetition and Practice

Once a restorative care activity is initiated, it is very important for older adults to have the opportunity to repeat this activity and practice performance. Older adults need to practice their self-care skills and thereby gain confidence in performance. The common expression "use it or lose it" comes to mind. As older adults master the various components of a self-care activity, they will need to practice those skills regularly. Communication and coordination among the nursing staff will ensure consistency in care practices. Inconsistencies among staff practices can be confusing for residents and can affect their desire and willingness to engage in self-care (see appendix).

Once a restorative care activity is mastered, the individual can progress to a higher level of performance. As mastery of various components of self-care skills occurs, new goals should be established. Ultimately, the goal of restorative care is to maintain the older individual at his or her highest level of function. When an older adult's performance reaches a plateau, goals should be directed toward maintaining the highest level of function reached. Caregiving practices need to ensure that self-performance is maintained.

RESTORATIVE CARE ACTIVITIES

Restorative activities can be general or task specific. Both types of activities are useful and contribute to the individual's ability to attain or maintain self-care skills. Tossing and catching a ball or resistive exercises such as lifting weights are general activities. These types of activities can improve strength, muscle tone, endurance, and balance, and may affect function (Baum, Jarjoura, Polen, Faur, & Ruteck, 2003; Evans, 1995; Fiatarone et al., 1994; Hagen, Armstrong-Esther, & Sandilands, 2003; Lazowski et al., 1999; Morris et al., 1999; Schnelle, Alessi et al., 2002). Baum and colleagues (2003) demonstrated that an exercise intervention, which included range of motion, elastic resistance bands, and soft weights, improved long-term care residents' ability to stand, balance, and perform physical tasks.

Task-specific activities, such as skill practice in using a sliding board or using an overhead trapeze bar to transfer from the bed to a chair, are targeted at improving specific aspects of function (Beck et al., 1997; Mulrow et al., 1994; Przybylski et al., 1996; Rogers et al., 1999; Tappen, 1994). Task-specific interventions usually combine an appropriate level and amount of staff assistance and specific strategies targeted at the cognitive ability and the functional deficits of the resident. Blair (1999) demonstrated that staffing training on topics such as determinants of dependency, behavior management, behavioral strategies, and goal attainment improved self-care performance and self-esteem among nursing home residents.

Restorative activities can be provided in either one-on-one sessions or group sessions. Tappen (1994) found that a 20-week (5 days per week) functional skill-training group intervention that focused on regaining function in the basic ADLs resulted in a significant improvement in self-maintenance (from major to moderate assistance or from moderate to minor assistance) and reductions in the amount of assistance provided to elderly nursing home residents who participated in the skill training class. Schnelle, Alessi, and colleagues (2002) demonstrated that a one-on-one intervention that encouraged nursing home residents to walk (if non-ambulatory, wheel), to repeat sit to stands at each 2-hour toileting episode, and to participate in a daily episode of upper body resistance training significantly maintained or improved residents' performance.

Finally, restorative activities can be planned or unplanned. Regularly scheduled skill practice sessions are the most common type of restorative activity, but staff members should look for unplanned opportunities to promote self-care. Seasonal events or recreational activities may provide opportunities for older adults to practice self-care skills. For example, transfer skills may be used in getting in and out of a car or van to take a trip to the mall or a baseball game. Participating in leisure activities such as bowling, dart throwing, ring toss, basketball toss, and horseshoes provides older adults with the opportunity to use upper body muscles and engage in coordination of movements that are needed to complete various ADLs.

SELF-CARE SKILLS

Self-care can be accomplished by using assistive techniques and devices that augment older adults' physical, psychological, or social limitations (Remsburg, 1999b). In general, restorative care should begin with observations of what the older adult can do. The environment should be modified to enhance self-care abilities, should be provided appropriate assistive devices, and verbal and physical prompts should be used. Modeling or demonstrating the self-care activity will assist some older adults, and they should be provided with positive feedback. Progress in meeting goals should be measured periodically. Once a goal is achieved, new goals should be established.

Residents should be prepared for participation in the restorative activity. Privacy should be provided, and the activity should be explained to the resident. Eyeglasses and hearing devices should be worn, and dentures should be in place. Residents should be toileted and, if indicated, analgesic medications should be taken. Residents should be positioned properly and monitored for fatigue. Caregivers should be encouraged to adopt a process-oriented approach rather than a task-oriented approach. How the self-care task is accomplished is as important as completing the task. It is essential to understand each functional skill and provide the appropriate techniques and devices to help the older individual perform each skill.

PERFORMANCE OF FUNCTIONAL SKILLS

Mobility

Mobility is integral to all self-care activities. Upper body mobility is needed for eating, bathing, grooming, dressing, and toileting. Lower body mobility is needed for toileting, transfers, ambulation, and locomotion. Interventions to maintain mobility among long-term care residents are effective (Koroknay, Werner, Cohen-Mansfield, Braun, 1995; MacRae et al., 1996; Schnelle, MacRae, Ouslander, Simmons, & Nitta, 1995; Tappen, Roach, Applegate, & Stowell, 2000). Tappen and colleagues (2000) found that nursing home residents with Alzheimer's disease who participated in an intervention that combined assisted walking with conversation for 30 minutes 3 times per week over a 16-week period maintained their functional mobility; and the use of conversation improved compliance with the intervention

Knowledge and skills needed for restorative mobility care include positioning, range of motion, transfers, and ambulation (Axelrod, 1999). Understanding of conditions and diseases that cause mobility impairments will assist restorative care providers in establishing appropriate restorative mobility goals and activities. For example, mobility activities used for progressive neurodegenerative diseases such as amyotrophic lateral sclerosis (ALS or Lou Gehrig's Disease) or multiple sclerosis will differ from activities used for residents with osteoarthritis or hemiplegia from cerebrovascular accidents.

Proper positioning and timely repositioning of residents with mobility impairments such as coma, paralysis, contractures, dystonia, dyskinesia, and neuropathies can prevent contractures, skin breakdown, aspiration, and injuries. Assistive devices such as splints, hand cones, and trochanter rolls can compensate for loss of muscle tone and spasticity. Residents who are able should be encouraged to participate in repositioning activities, such as rolling from side to side. Awareness of positions that are contraindicated, such as leg adduction after hip replacement, is imperative. Proper support of limbs during repositioning prevents stress and injury and minimizes pain to joints. Protecting bony prominences with elbow and heel protectors will prevent skin friction and breakdown.

Range of motion (ROM) exercises are used to preserve normal joint function, maintain or improve muscle strength and endurance, and prevent contractures. These exercises can be done alone or in conjunction with other self-care activities such as bathing and positioning. Exercise and recreational activities that involve movement, such as tai chi, ball tosses, bowling, and gardening, also promote and maintain joint mobility.

ROM exercises can be either passive or active. Passive ROM is performed by the restorative care provider and usually is used when the resident is unable to perform these activities. Sometimes, however, a resident can be taught to perform passive ROM exercises. A resident with left-side paresis could perform ROM on the impaired left arm with the unaffected right arm. The resident can perform active ROM exercises independently or with help from a caregiver. Families can be taught how to do ROM exercises, which provides them an active way to be involved in caring for their loved one. Active ROM can be used to increase circulation, increase sensory awareness and joint motion, improve or maintain coordination and muscle strength, and in some cases improve cardiovascular and lung function.

Initiation of any type of restorative mobility program, including ROM, should begin slowly, increasing repetition of motion over time. Excessive repetitions or overextension of normal joint function can result in inflammation and pain, conditions that can lead to an older adult's unwillingness to continue with the exercise program. For individuals with painful medical conditions such as arthritis or joint replacement, administration of analgesic medications 30 to 60 minutes before initiating ROM can prevent unnecessary pain and promote joint mobility. Restorative care providers should be alert for muscle spasms and cramps, which often can be managed with gentle pressure and massage.

Transfer Techniques

Safe and efficient transfer, the movement of an individual from one surface to another, depends on the interaction of the individual's physical abilities, perceptual capacity, and use of assistive equipment, appropriate techniques, and planning. An older adult can transfer independently or with the assistance of one or more caregivers. Transfers can be accomplished using simple techniques or assistive devices or mechanical lifts. Assistive transfer devices include gait belts, sliding boards, overhead trapeze bars, grab bars, side rails, and handrails (Allen, Jackson, Marsden, McLellan, & Gore, 2002; Garg, Owen, Beller, & Banaag, 1991; Zhuang, Stobbe, Collins, Hsiao, & Hobbs, 1999; 2000). Ergonomic principles, that is, proper body mechanics and lifting techniques, should be observed when assisting residents in transfers (Galensky, Waters, & Malit, 2001; Garg, Owen, &

Carlson, 1992; Owen, Keene, & Olson, 2002). Improper lifting techniques and incorrect use of assistive devices can result in injury to both the caregiver and the older adult (Daynard et al., 2001; Lynch, & Freund, 2000; Nelson, Lloyd, Menzel, Gross, 2003; Yassi et al., 2001). Basic principles to follow include using good posture; bending at the knee instead of the back; maintaining a wide stance; moving close to the object or person before lifting; pushing, pulling, or rolling heavy objects whenever possible instead of lifting; and turning by moving feet instead of twisting the back.

Whenever possible, older adults should be encouraged to participate in the transfer. If the older individual can participate, is not totally dependent, and is not obese, transfers can often be accomplished with physical assistance and coaching from the caregiver using assistive devices such a gait belt or a sliding board. For older adults who are unable to participate or who are obese, the use of mechanical lifting devices is recommended. Sit-to-stand lifts are useful for older adults with intact upper body mobility. Total body lifts are useful for large or obese individuals and those who have limited upper and lower body mobility. The use of mechanical lifting devices can be frightening for some older adults. They need explanations about the lifting and reassurance during the transfer and should never be left alone while suspended by a mechanical lifting device.

Ambulation

Ambulation refers to the act of walking, either independently or with the assistance of a device or caregiver. Safe ambulation requires balance, strength, and coordination. Restorative ambulation activities and assistive devices are designed to improve or augment deficits in balance, strength, and coordination.

Walking interventions designed to maintain or improve ambulation among nursing home residents are effective (Koroknay et al., 1995; MacRae et al., 1996; Schnelle, MacRae et al., 1995; Tappen et al., 2000). The first step in providing restorative ambulation care is establishing and maintaining a safe environment, free of obstacles and hazards such as TV cords or slippery floors. Adequate lighting and elimination of glare are important. Properly fitting shoes with nonslip soles and assistive devices such as canes or walkers adjusted to the appropriate height are important. Ambulation assistive devices include braces, knee immobilizers, prosthetic devices, shoe lifts, crutches, canes, and walkers. Canes are used to compensate for impaired balance and improve stability. Walkers are used to provide support and stability for individuals who have leg weakness or more severe balance problems, and who are able to weight bear on one leg.

Awareness of fatigue is critical. The caregiver should be alert to signs of fatigue and anticipate the need to rest. A wheelchair or chair should be available for older adults who become fatigued. The use of a gait belt is recommended and can be used to lower the individual to the floor if weakness or instability occurs.

Older adults involved in restorative ambulation programs should be assessed for fall risk. Factors associated with falls include sensory impairments, orthostatic hypotension, cardiac arrhythmias, confusion, incontinence, and use of antihypertensive, diuretic, hypoglycemic, and psychotropic medications. As older individuals gain mobility and confidence, they may overestimate their abilities and attempt ambulation on their own. They need to be made aware of their abilities and limitations. Premature attempts to ambulate or transfer independently can result in injury.

Locomotion

In addition to regaining or maintaining mobility, restorative care often involves improving older adults' locomotion abilities. Locomotion refers to the ability to move around the environment, from room to room or floor to floor. Wheelchairs are frequently used to augment locomotion deficits. Wheelchairs promote older adults' independence and may enhance their abilities to do other self-care activities such as toileting (Pawlson, Goodwin, & Keith, 1986). However, wheelchairs can also promote dependence. Older adults in wheelchairs are often viewed as immobile and therefore treated as immobile, and, unfortunately, wheelchairs may accelerate mobility dependence (Simmons, Schnelle, MacRae, & Ouslander, 1995). Older adults in wheelchairs should be encouraged to wheel themselves, thus promoting and preserving upper body strength and mobility. Restorative care for older adults in wheelchairs should include exercise of lower extremities to maintain muscle tone and strength and to preserve transfer abilities. It is essential that older adults who can walk be encouraged and assisted to do so.

Eating

The ability to feed oneself and to enjoy food are important for quality of life and can affect feelings of dignity and self-worth. Improving or maintaining self-feeding skills promotes independence, enhances dignity, and can improve hydration and nutritional status. Studies in nursing homes and home settings indicate numerous preventable and reversible causes of poor food consumption, including unappetizing food and use of restrictive diets, inappropriate assistance from staff, and suboptimal dining environments (Amella, 1998; Blaum, Fries, Fiatarone, 1995; Kayser-Jones, 1996; 1997; Kayser-Jones & Schell, 1997a and b; Morley & Kraenzle, 1994; Morley & Silver, 1995).

Several studies suggest that modifications of food service, dining environment, and mealtime feeding assistance may improve quantity and quality of food consumption in older adults (Crogan & Shultz, 2000; Kayser-Jones, 1996; 1997; Kayser-Jones & Schell, 1997; Remsburg, Luking et al., 2001; Steele, Greenwood, Ens, Robertson, Seidman-Carlson, 1997). Improving the taste of the food, using decentralized bulk-food portioning, playing music during mealtimes, creating a family-style dining room, and providing personalized feeding assistance have been shown to increase food intake (Elmstahl, Blabolil, Fex, Kuller, Steen, 1987; Mathey, Siebelink, de Graaf, & Van Staveren, 2001; Mathey, Vanneste, de Graaf, de Groot, & van Staveren, 2001; Ragneskog, Brane, Karlsson, & Kihlgren, 1996; Ragneskog, Kihlgren, Karlsson, & Norberg, 1996; Shatenstein, Ska, & Ferland, 2001; Remsburg et al. 2001; Simmons et al., 2001). Interventions to improve self-feeding and food consumption among older adults are effective (Lange-Alberts & Shott, 1994; Osborn & Marshall, 1993; Simmons, Alessi, & Schnelle, 2001; Simmons, Osterweil & Schnelle, 2001; Van Ort & Phillips, 1995). These interventions include use of one-on-one feeding assistance, verbal prompts, food preference, touch and verbal cuing, and a system of least prompts.

Self-feeding can be accomplished by using assistive devices and providing the appropriate type and level of assistance (Remsburg, 1999a). Independence in feeding can be enhanced by proper positioning, making sure dentures are in place, and attending to oral hygiene and dental conditions such as painful lesions or broken teeth, and identifying swallowing disorders.

Self-feeding can also be enhanced by providing tasty, seasoned food that the individual likes, maintaining the appropriate food temperature, and providing the texture and consistency of food that matches the individual's chewing abilities. For some older adults, assistance with meal setup, such as, removing drink covers, pouring milk into a glass, buttering bread, or chopping food, is all that is needed.

Assistive feeding devices are designed to augment impairments such as inability to grasp small objects, unsteady or uncoordinated hand movement, and swallowing or chewing problems. Assistive devices used for self-feeding include specialty utensils, sip cups, sectioned plates, and plate guards. For older adults with cognitive impairment, simple verbal prompts and cuing may promote self-feeding. Some older adults may need assistance with scooping or spearing food, but once food is placed on the spoon or fork they are able to feed themselves. For those who lose the ability to use utensils, finger foods such as sandwiches, cheese sticks, breakfast bars, gelatin squares, fish sticks, chicken nuggets, and other food items that do not require use of utensils can promote self-feeding.

Creating a pleasant dining atmosphere can also enhance mealtime food consumption. Ragneskog and colleagues (Ragneskog, Brane et al., 1996; Rageskog, Kihlgren et al., 1996) found that both residents and staff were positively influenced by music played at mealtimes, and on days music was played, staff served residents more food and residents spent more time eating.

Observational tools can be used to assess the quality of assistance provided by feeding assisters. Simmons, Babineau, Garcia, and Schnelle (2002) developed a standardized feeding assistance observational protocol that consists of four feeding assistance care quality indicators (QIs) that can be used to identify caregiver ability to (1) accurately identify residents with low oral food and fluid intake during mealtime; (2) provide feeding assistance to at-risk residents during mealtime; (3) provide feeding assistance to residents identified as requiring staff assistance to eat; and (4) provide verbal prompts to residents who receive physical assistance at mealtimes. The Quality of Feeding Assistance Assessment, another observational tool, can be used to assess assistants' feeding skills and to train staff to provide more individualized assistance (Table 4.4).

Table 4.4   Quality of Feeding Assistance Assessment

Time feeding started:_____   Time feeding ended:_____

Diet order:_____

What type of assistance does the resident require: *Circle the appropriate response.*

1) **No helper: Complete independence**—Resident eats from a dish, while managing all consistencies of food, drinks, from a cup or glass, with the meal presented in the customary manner on a table or tray. The resident uses a spoon or fork to bring food to mouth; food is chewed and swallowed.

2) **No helper: Modified independence**—Resident requires an adaptive or assistive device such as a long straw, spork, rocking knife; requires more than a reasonable time to eat; or requires modified food consistency or blenderized food, or there are safety considerations.

3) **Helper: Supervision or setup**—Resident requires supervision (e.g., standing by, cueing, or coaxing) or setup, or another person is required to open containers, cut meats, butter bread, or pour liquids.

4) **Helper: Minimal contact assistance**—Resident performs 75% or more of eating tasks.

5) **Helper: Moderate assistance**—Resident performs 50–74% of eating tasks.

6) **Helper: Maximal assistance**—Resident performs 25–49% of eating tasks.

7) **Helper: Total assistance**—Resident performs less than 25% of eating tasks.

Preparation of the Environment	Never	Occasionally	Often	Always	Not Applicable	Comments
Eliminates distractions (turns off TV)						
Assists resident to dining room or prepares dining place in resident's room (clears off over-bed table and places tray/food within reach)						
Eliminates noxious stimuli (bedpan, urinal), pulls bedside curtains						
Groups residents who have similar assistive or social needs (minimal assists together, total assists together)						
Preparation of the Resident	Never	Occasionally	Almost Always	Always	Not Applicable	Comments
Eyeglasses/assistive hearing device (if applicable)						
Dentures (if applicable)						
Protective garment (bib) (if applicable)						
Seated position (comfortable, feet on floor, back supported)						
Proper table height (not too high not too low)						
Able to reach plate						
Food and Implements	Never	Occasionally	Almost Always	Always	Not Applicable	Comments
Checks diet order if uncertain						
Food placed within reach (in field of view)						
Food unobstructed (lids off, condiments open, straws open)						
Minimizes obstacles (take food off tray and place on table)						
Cuts food into appropriate size pieces (if that's all the assistance the resident needs)						
Seasons food appropriately (e.g., salts food if patient can have salt, uses food enhancer if resident can't have salt)						
Obtains assistive feeding device and assists resident in appropriate use of device						
Modifies the feeding implements to facilitate self-feeding (puts straw in cup, puts soup in a cup, puts entrée in a bowl)						

(continued)

Table 4.4   *Continued*

Food and Implements (*cont.*)	Never	Occasionally	Almost Always	Always	Not Applicable	Comments
Monitors resident (if resident does not eat or eats very little, inquires why and offers substitutions)						
Monitors for fatigue and assists when appropriate						
Feeding Assistance Provided	Never	Occasionally	Almost Always	Always	Not Applicable	Comments
Sits down with resident						
Observes resident for evidence of self-feeding behaviors						
First offers verbal coaching: "Mrs. White, take a biteof potatoes"						
Then offers minimal physical assistance						
Loads the fork/spoon and places in resident's hand, places finger food in hand, places cup in hand						
Pantomimes eating						
Offers praise and positive feedback when task is accomplished						
Uses finger food (or makes food into finger food, e.g., makes a sandwich, cuts meat, and offers pieces)						
Encourages resident to consume beverages						
Follows specified feeding plan (e.g., provides correct food texture—pureed or chopped, care plan states "add milk to pureed foods to enhance texture for swallowing")						
Informs resident of food being offered						
Loads spoon or fork with appropriate amount of food (what the resident is able to handle)						
Offers beverage after several bites						
Performs end of meal hygiene (wipes mouth, hands, removes bibs, cleans up spills)						
Feeding Style	Never	Occasionally	Almost Always	Always	Not Applicable	Comments
Offers all foods on tray/plate						
Attempts to obtain and offer substitutions						
Attempts to enhance food quality (adds condiments, gravy, heats food, adds ice to beverage)						
Waits a few minutes and then offers food again						
Indiscriminant mixing of foods						
Offers liquid supplement before using assistive techniques described above						
Rushes resident						
Forces food or beverage into resident's mouth						
Removes tray/food before resident is finished						
Removes tray/serving dishes but leaves food items for resident to eat						

Other Comments/Observations:

Bathing

Bathing is a personal and private activity. Inability to bathe can lead to feelings of inadequacy and embarrassment. For older adults with cognitive impairment, bathing can be a frightening and confusing experience, and can therefore lead to disruptive or resistive behavior. Promoting independence in bathing can improve hygiene and restore dignity. Bathing or showering also can be soothing and relaxing for older adults.

Most studies of bathing of older adults are designed to reduce disruptive or aggressive behaviors (Barrick, Rader, Hoeffer, & Sloane, 2001; Hoeffer, Rader, McKenzie, Lavelle, & Stewart, 1997; Kovach & Meyer-Arnold, 1997; Maxfield, Lewis, & Cannon, 1996; Miller, 1997; Sloane et al., 1995). With training and guidance from nurses, nursing assistants can learn to effectively assist older adults with dementia in bathing. Creating a calm and soothing atmosphere, creating a pleasant bath/shower room environment, and using a calm, unrushed approach are key strategies for bathing older adults with dementia.

Independence in bathing can be accomplished by using assistive devices and providing the appropriate type and level of assistance (Remsburg, 1999a). Bathing can occur in the privacy of the older adult's room, a bathroom, or a shower or tub room. Providing and maintaining privacy can reduce embarrassment; maintaining a warm room temperature can promote comfort. Adding plants, curtains, wallpaper, warm wall colors, pictures and eliminating unsightly supplies and nonbathing equipment can enhance the appearance of the bathroom and reduce fear associated with bathing (Kraker & Vajdik, 1997; Martin, 1998; Rader, Lavelle, Hoeffer, & McKenzie, 1996). When showers and tub rooms are used, safety precautions such as rubber floor mats, grab bars, and bath stools can prevent bath time falls and injuries. Older adults should never be left alone in the tub or shower. With older adults for whom a tub bath or shower is extremely stressful or contraindicated, towel baths and waterless disposable bath products can be used (Birch & Coggins, 2003; Skewes, 1997).

Independence in bathing can often be enhanced by assembling and making bathing supplies accessible to the older individual. Many older adults are able to perform some parts of the bath, such as wash their face or upper torso. It is important, therefore, to encourage them to do any part of the bath they are able to perform.

Some older individuals may need verbal cues and prompts, and some may need gentle physical support. Gently guiding a hand holding a washcloth to the face may be sufficient for some older adults to initiate bathing activities. Other individuals may need visual cues such as modeling or demonstration of the activity.

Assistive devices such as sponges, handled sponges, wash mittens, disposable wipes, soap dispensers, or soap on a rope can be used to promote self-bathing. For older adults who have difficulty handling soap and water, wet, and warmed washcloths can be placed in a plastic bag. For individuals with difficulty reaching lower extremities, wet, warm and soaped towels can be used. By holding both ends of the towel, the older adult can pull the towel back and forth over various body parts. A wet and warmed towel can be used to wipe away soap and a dry towel can be used for drying wet skin. Disposable bathing products can also be used.

The Caregiver Behavior Checklist may be a useful tool to assess caregivers' bathing skills (Barrick et al., 2001). This 11-item instrument can be used to assess a caregiver's verbal and nonverbal communication, task presentation style, and independence-promoting behaviors (Table 4.5). Specific interventions can then be implemented to facilitate self-care activities.

Grooming

Improving self-grooming skills promotes independence, improves hygiene, and preserves dignity. Maintaining the ability to attend to personal hygiene and appearance can affect an older adult's self-esteem, desire to participate in social activities, and general sense of well-being. Specific interventions designed to improve older adults' self-grooming abilities have been noted to be effective (Blair, 1999; Lim, 2003; Pyle, Massie, & Nelson, 1998; Rogers et al., 1999, Tappen, 1994). Lim (2003) used systematic prompting and social reinforcement to provide nursing home residents with dementia a series of one-step commands to guide their face-washing, tooth-brushing, and hair-combing. Residents participating in the intervention demonstrated significant increases in grooming independence. Other interventions include behavior management and mutual goal setting, nursing assistant training, skill elicitation (determining task skills retained and structuring the physical and social environment to facilitate use of the skills), and functional skill training.

Table 4.5 Caregiver Behavior Checklist

Name of caregiver: _____ Person being bathed: _____ Date of bath: _____

Verbal Communication	Never	Almost Never	Occasionally	Often	Almost Always	Always
Praises resident	1	2	3	4	5	6
Uses a calm voice	1	2	3	4	5	6
Speaks respectfully	1	2	3	4	5	6
Expresses concern/interest	1	2	3	4	5	6
Speaks directly to resident	1	2	3	4	5	6
Task Presentation						
Prepares resident for the task	1	2	3	4	5	6
Bathes at a pace appropriate for this resident	1	2	3	4	5	6
Nonverbal Communication						
Gently touches resident	1	2	3	4	5	6
Is flexible with the bathing routine	1	2	3	4	5	6
Makes eye contact with the resident	1	2	3	4	5	6
Independence (assess if appropriate)						
Encourages independence	1	2	3	4	5	6

TOTAL: _____

Using assistive devices and providing the appropriate type and level of assistance can enhance grooming independence (Remsburg, 1999a). Assembling and making grooming supplies accessible can enhance self-grooming ability. Providing privacy during restorative grooming activities will help prevent embarrassment. The use of assistive devices such as a built-up comb, hairbrush, toothbrush, or razor; electric razor or toothbrush; or stationary fingernail brushes can enhance self-grooming abilities. A large mirror and adequate lighting should be provided. Glasses and hearing devices should be worn. Older adults should be encouraged to complete any part of the grooming activities they are able to complete.

Applying makeup, aftershave lotion, and cologne should be encouraged. Applying moisture lotion can prevent dry skin, and applying sunscreen can prevent sunburn if outdoor activities are planned. Some older adults may need simple verbal prompts or cues, and some may need physical cues such as guiding their hand holding the comb to their head to comb the hair. Other older individuals may benefit from modeling and demonstration.

Dressing

Personal appearance is also important for self-esteem and can affect older adults' desire to participate in so-cial activities such as visiting with family or friends, eating in the dining room, or participating in recreational activities. Improving self-dressing skills can promote independence and dignity. Nursing assistants can learn to implement strategies designed to promote independence in dressing among older adults (Beck et al., 1997; Engelman et al., 2002; Rogers et al., 1999; Tappen, 1994).

Dressing independence can be accomplished by using assistive devices and providing the appropriate type and level of assistance (Remsburg, 1999a). Many older individuals can perform self-dressing when clothes and shoes are placed within reach. Clothing appropriate for age, gender, and season should be provided. Clothes should be clean and fit well. Shoes should fit properly, with thin nonskid soles and low heels (Lord & Bashford, 1996; Robbins, Gouw, & McClaran, 1992). A mirror should be available for the older adult to use as a visual aid. Simple modifications to clothing, such as adding Velcro to shirts or pants or using clothes that are slightly oversized, can promote self-dressing (Cole, 1992).

Common assistive dressing devices include reachers, button fasteners, zipper pulls, stocking aids, long-handled shoehorns, and step stools. Older individuals should be instructed on the optimal sequencing for donning clothes, such as dressing weak or impaired limbs first. Donning a bra can be particularly challenging for some women, who can be instructed to fasten the clasp first, place arms through the straps, and then pull the bra up over the breasts.

Some older adults will need only verbal prompts or cues, while others will need physical assistance, such as holding the shirt as the individual inserts his or her arm into the shirt sleeve. Demonstrations on donning various clothing items can be useful for some older adults. As with other self-care activities, older adults should be encouraged to participate in any part of the dressing activity that they are able to complete. Donning shoes can be facilitated by using a foot stool, a reacher, or slide-on shoes.

For older adults with cognitive impairment, a dressing assessment guide may be useful in assessing individuals' self-dressing abilities (Heacock, Beck, Souder, & Mercer, 1997). The assessment is designed to identify (1) cognitive assets and deficits such as attention, voluntary motor actions, fine and gross motor skills, visual organization and perception, language ability, and functional skills needed in dressing; and (2) remaining functional capacities. This tool can be used to develop individualized clinical interventions for persons with dementia. See Table 4.6 for quidelines for a group grooming and dressing class.

Toileting

Self-toileting is important for maintaining self-esteem, continence, and hygiene, and for preventing skin breakdown. Interventions and strategies to promote toileting and prevent incontinence demonstrate that caregiver behaviors significantly influence toileting outcomes (Burgio et al., 1994; Colling, Ouslander, Hadley, Eisch, & Campbell, 1992; Engel et al., 1990; Glenn, 2003; Hu et al., 1989; Lekan-Rutledge, 2000; Rogers et al., 1999; Schnelle, 1990; Schnelle, MacRae et al., 1995; Schnelle, Newman et al., 1993; Tappen, 1994).

Restorative toilet activities are designed to promote independence, prevent incontinence, and maintain proper bladder and bowel function. Older adults who are unable to toilet themselves, who soil themselves, or who are forced to wear adult protective pads may feel ashamed and embarrassed. Wearing "adult diapers" can be demeaning and lead to total dependency. Declines in toileting ability can lead to declines in mobility and other self-care activities.

Using assistive devices and providing the appropriate type and level of assistance can enhance toileting

Table 4.6 Recommendations for Grooming and Dressing Classes

Candidates for grooming classes are those who have been identified as in need of skills training, those who have a potential for increased grooming function, or those who will not be able to increase function but will still gain sensory stimulation and pride in their appearance.

Factors to Consider
1. Classes need to meet individual grooming goals whether they be washing hands or face, combing hair, applying makeup, working with buttons, tying shoes.
2. Make each class specific to an individual task; do not try to do too much at once.
3. Make the tasks easy to adapt to each resident's ability.
4. Sales representatives of various products, Avon, Mary Kay, etc., are usually glad to donate items for the class, or you can have a grooming class fundraising event to solicit items for use.
5. Regular attendees may like to have their own cosmetic bag of items needed for class.
6. Use colors, textures, and smells.
7. Dressing is important; teach each aspect in a single class.
8. Plan a special fashion show after a few months of classes.
9. Use of mirrors is important; make sure everyone can use one.
10. Staff involvement is important not only during the class but afterward to provide compliments.
11. Get the hairdresser to do demonstrations, using a model.
12. Let residents select colors of nail polish, lipstick, hair bows, etc.
13. Don't forget the men for shaving, special dressing, and shoes.
14. Be sure to include confused residents in the group; you may need to divide into several groups that meet regularly together.

independence (Remsburg, 1999a). Toileting is a private activity, and most residents have long-standing bladder and bowel habits. A major challenge for the restorative care providers is providing the appropriate level of assistance while ensuring privacy.

Restoring self-toileting activities should include an assessment of the older adult's nutritional intake and hydration. Consuming adequate fluids and bulk-containing foods promotes normal bladder and bowel function. Before beginning restorative toileting activities, residents with episodes of incontinence should have a thorough physical and medical evaluation. Reversible causes of incontinence, such as urinary tract infections or constipation, should be treated. Working with the individual's primary health care provider to determine the type of incontinence (e.g., urge, stress, or combination) will allow caregivers to develop the most appropriate and effective toileting strategies.

Monitoring the older individual's toileting routine over a 3-day period can help establish an appropriate toileting schedule. Reminders and assistance from the restorative care provider at these times can improve continence and toileting self-care. Assistive devices such as bedside commodes, raised toilet seats, grab bars, fracture bedpans, urinals, toilet tissue, and water-free hand cleansers can be used to increase self-toileting.

Prompted voiding techniques and bladder retraining can be useful as well (Glenn, 2003; Schnelle, 1990). Prompted voiding combines routinely scheduled toileting times and positive reinforcement by caregivers when elimination occurs to retrain residents to void at the regularly scheduled times. Bladder retraining can be effective for older individuals recovering from conditions that affect the ability to perceive or control bladder filling and emptying, such as stroke or abdominal surgery. Bladder retraining involves gradually extending the length of time between regularly scheduled toileting episodes. Through practice, older individuals can increase the length of time between toileting episodes (Glen, 2003).

Restorative toileting interventions can be time consuming and labor intensive, and without organizational support and resources continence programs often fail (Schnelle, Kapur et al., 2003; Smith, 1998). Supervision and quality monitoring to ensure caregiver adherence to individualized toileting programs will improve toileting outcomes.

Exercise

The benefits of exercise are well known and include muscle strength and tone, balance and agility, joint mobility, cardiovascular capacity, mood, and well-being. Recent studies demonstrate that even very frail and functionally impaired older adults can benefit from exercise (Baum et al., 2003; Evans, 1995; 1999; Fiatarone et al., 1994; Lazowski et al., 1999; Li et al., 2001; Morris et al., 1999; Taggart, 2002; Nowalk, Predergast, Bayles, D'Amico, & Colvin, 2001). Lazowski and colleagues (1999) used nursing aides and volunteers who completed a physical activity workshop to conduct group exercise classes for 45 minutes three times per week. Classes included progressive strengthening exercises using soft weights and elastic bands, balance and flexibility exercises, and walking. Nursing home residents participating in the intervention had significant improvements in mobility, balance, flexibility, and knee and hip strength. Taggert (2002) demonstrated improvements in balance and functional mobility and decreases in fear of falling scores for older women in retirement communities participating in Tai chi 2 days per week.

Older adults respond well to resistive training, high-intensity progressive resistance using weights or equipment, and Tai chi, an ancient Chinese martial art consisting of a series of slow but continuous movements of every body part. Resistance training can be accomplished by using hand and leg weights, resistive elastic bands, or specialized exercise equipment. Gradual increase of the weight of the resistance and the number of repetitions improves endurance and muscle strength and tone. Tai chi involves repetitions of a series of movements of the head, eyes, arms, hands, body, legs, and feet done in coordination with the mind and respiration. Tai chi movements incorporate elements of muscle strengthening, balance, and postural alignment (Wu, 2002).

As with younger adults, older adults' compliance with exercise interventions is often difficult to sustain (Nowalk et al., 2000). Exercise regimens that incorporate social and recreational features are associated with better compliance (Hagen et al., 2003; Mathews, Clair, Kosloski 2001; Tappen et al., 2000). Music and conversation during exercise are effective strategies for maintaining exercise compliance, as are exercise programs that can be easily incorporated into daily activities, such as those shown in Table 4.7. Ideas for group activities that involve movement are described in Table 4.8. Other strategies to motivate older adults to engage in exercise and other restorative activities can be found in chapter 5.

ENSURING SUCCESS IN RESTORATIVE CARE ACTIVITIES

Key elements to successful provision of restorative care include the involvement of the older adult, family, and other caregivers; organizational support if the individual is institutionalized; education and training of all caregivers; supervision and communication; and flexibility and creativity in developing restorative activities. For restorative care to be successful, the individual, his or her family, and caregivers need to be involved in establishing the restorative goal and the

Table 4.7   Exercise Program for Bedbound, Nonambulatory, and Ambulatory Older Adults

Standing Exercises

Patient must be able to stand independently (support of a walker/cane is allowable).

Head turns—Stand using a stable surface for balance or support.
Look over the right shoulder; count to 5.
Look over the left shoulder; count to 5.
Repeat the sequence 5 times.

Head tilts—Stand using a stable surface for balance and support.
While looking forward, tilt head to the right shoulder; count to 5.
While looking forward, tilt head to the left shoulder; count to 5.
Repeat the sequence 5 times.

"I don't know's"—Stand using a stable surface for balance and support.
Look forward and shrug shoulders up to ears; count to 5.
Lower shoulders to starting position; count to 5.
Repeat sequence 5 times.

Shoulder rolls—Stand using a stable surface for balance and support.
Look forward; roll both shoulders forward.
Repeat 5 times.
Look forward; roll both shoulders backward.
Repeat 5 times.

Airplanes—Stand using a stable surface for balance and support.
Hold onto a stable surface with one hand.
Hold other arm straight out to the front.
Circle straight arm 5 times to the right and 5 times to the left.
Repeat the sequence using the other arm.
(If able, can do both arms at the same time.)

Tea pot side bends—Stand using a stable surface for balance and support.
Hold stable surface with one hand.
Place the other arm above your head (slightly bent).
Bend sideways at the waist away from the raised arm.
Return to the starting position.
Repeat 5 times to one side then switch arms and repeat sequence to the other side.
Modification for those who cannot successfully reach arm above head:
Place hand on the head to do the side bend.

Bow to the queen—Stand using a stable surface for balance and support.
Stand facing a stable surface, or if able stand with the stable surface at your side and hold with one hand.
Keep legs and back as straight as possible.
Bend forward at the hip (do not go past 90 degrees).
Count to 5.
Return to starting position.
Repeat 5 times.

On your mark, get set, go—Stand using a stable surface for balance and support.
Place left foot 12–24 inches behind the right foot.
Keep both feet flat on the floor.
Slightly bend the right knee, keeping left leg as straight as possible.
While looking forward, press upper body forward.
Count to 5.

Return to upright position.
Repeat 5 times, then switch feet and repeat 5 times with the left foot to the front.
These exercises may be done using light wrist weights/dumbbells, elastic exercise bands or no resistance at all.

Move the mountain—Stand facing a wall.
Place feet 12–18 inches away from the wall.
Place hands flat on the wall at shoulder height.
Keep both feet flat on the floor.
Bend both arms (about 90 degrees).
Straighten arms and return to starting position.
Repeat up to 10 times.
This exercise is *not* recommended for those with severe shoulder, elbow, or wrist problems causing severe pain or limited range of motion..

Popeye exercise—Stand with stable surface within reach.
Hold right arm straight down at the side.
Keep elbow glued to the waist.
Palm facing forward.
Bend elbow.
Lift palm up to the shoulder.
Return to the starting position.
Repeat up to 10 times with the right arm.
Switch to the left arm and repeat up to 10 times.
A weight or elastic exercise band may be used to make the exercise a little more difficult.

Hugs—Stand with stable surface within reach.
Hold slightly bent arms horizontally out to your sides.
Palms face each other.
Bring arms in toward the center and give yourself a hug.
Count to 5.
Open arms out to the side (keeping them slightly bent).
Repeat the sequence up to 10 times.
A weight may be held in each hand to make the exercise a little more difficult.

Fly away wings—Stand with stable surface within reach.
Hold both arms straight down at the sides with palms facing your thighs.
Raise both arms out to the side.
Stop at shoulder height.
Count to 5.
Lower to starting position.
Repeat sequence up to 10 times.
Hold a weight in each hand to make the exercise a little more difficult.

Kick the dog—Stand facing a stable surface for balance and support.
Keep the legs as straight as possible.
Lift one leg out to the side (about 10–12 inches), keeping toes facing forward.
Count to 5.
Return to starting position.
Repeat up to 10 times with one leg.
Repeat the sequence using the other leg.
A weight may be placed on the ankle to make the exercise a little harder. To make the exercise a little easier, have the patient touch the toes out to the side instead of lifting off the floor. *(continued)*

Table 4.7 *Continued*

Standing Exercises (*cont.*)

A kick in the butt—Stand facing a stable surface for balance and support.

> Keep support leg as straight as possible.
> Lift the other leg backward by bending the knee.
> Raise the foot about 12–18 inches above the floor.
> Count to 5.
> Return to starting position with both feet flat on the floor.
> Repeat up to 10 times.
> Repeat the sequence using the other leg.
>> A weight may be placed on the ankle of the "lifting" leg to make the exercise a little harder.

Ballerina—Stand facing a stable surface for balance and support.

> Stand with both feet flat and about 2–4 inches apart.
> Lift both heels about 2 inches off the floor.
> Count to 5.
> Lower both heels to the floor.
> Repeat the sequence up to 10 times.

Stand up and march—Stand facing a stable surface for balance and support, have a stable chair (with arms if possible) or a locked wheelchair directly behind the patient.

> Stand with feet a comfortable distance apart.
> Sit slowly into the chair with or without hand support.
> Count to 2.
> Stand as quickly and safely as possible (hands may be used if needed).
> Stand upright and begin marching in place 10 times.
> Stop marching and repeat the sequence up to 10 times.

Seated Exercises

Choose at least 2 exercises from each exercise group.
Patients should be independent sitting in a chair or wheelchair.

Head turns

> Look over the right shoulder; count to 5.
> Look over the left shoulder; count to 5.
> Repeat the sequence 5 times.

Head tilts

> While looking forward, tilt head to the right shoulder; count to 5.
> While looking forward, tilt head to the left shoulder; count to 5.
> Repeat the sequence 5 times.

"I don't know's"

> Look forward and shrug shoulders up to ears; count to 5.
> Lower shoulders to starting position; count to 5.
> Repeat sequence 5 times.

Shoulder rolls

> Look forward and roll both shoulders forward.
> Repeat 5 times.
> Look forward and roll both shoulders backward.
> Repeat 5 times.

Airplanes

> Hold onto a stable surface with one hand.
> Hold other arm straight out to the front.
> Circle straight arm 5 times to the right and 5 times to the left.
> Repeat the sequence using the other arm.
> (If able can do both arms at the same time.)

Teapot side bends—Sit in a chair or wheelchair with feet flat on the floor (if possible).

> Place one arm above your head (slightly bent).
> Bend sideways at the waist away from the raised arm.
> Return to the starting position.
> Repeat 5 times to one side, then switch arms and repeat sequence to the other side.
> Modification for those who cannot successfully reach arm above head:
>> Place hand on the head to do the side bend.
>> **CAUTION:** To prevent someone from falling out of the chair while doing side bends, always use a chair with arms.

Check those toes—Sit in a chair or wheelchair with feet flat on the floor.

> Lift toes up while keeping heels touching the floor.
> Count to 5.
> Lower toes to the floor.
> Repeat up to 10 times.

Show those toes—Sit in a chair or wheelchair.

> While keeping the left foot on the floor, lift the right foot until the right knee is as straight as possible.
> Point the toes forward, then pull the toes back to flex the foot.
> Repeat the point and flex 10 times.
> Lower the right foot to the floor.
> Repeat the sequence using the left foot.
> Now circle the right foot clockwise 5 times.
> Circle the right foot counterclockwise 5 times.
> Lower the right foot to the floor.
> Repeat the sequence using the left foot.
>> **Use caution when working with individuals with hip replacements or severe degeneration of the hip joint.**

Chair push Ups—Sit in a chair with arms or a wheelchair.

> Place hands securely on the arms of the chair.
> Raise hips about 2–6 inches by straightening the arms.
> Count to 2 (be sure the patient is breathing during the entire exercise).
> Slowly lower until arms are relaxed.
> Repeat up to 10 times.
>> **Use caution: this is a difficult exercise. The patients must not hold their breath at any time. Stop if chest, shoulder, neck, elbow, wrist, or hand pain occurs.**

Popeye exercise

> Hold right arm straight down at the side.
> Keep elbow glued to the waist.
> Palm facing forward.
> Bend elbow.
> Lift palm up to the shoulder.
> Return to the starting position.
> Repeat up to 10 times with the right arm.
> Switch to the left arm and repeat up to 10 times.
>> A weight or elastic exercise band may be used to make the exercise a little more difficult.

Hugs

> Hold slightly bent arms horizontally out to your sides.
> Palms face each other.
> Bring arms in toward the center and give yourself a hug.

Table 4.7   *Continued*

Count to 5.

Open arms out to the side (keeping them slightly bent).

Repeat the sequence up to 10 times.

A weight may be held in each hand to make the exercise a little more difficult.

Fly away wings

Hold both arms straight down at the sides with palms facing your thighs.

Raise both arms out to the side.

Stop at shoulder height.

Count to 5.

Lower to starting position.

Repeat sequence up to 10 times.

Scrub the countertop—Sit in a chair or wheelchair.

Hold arms as straight as possible out to the front.

Palms should face down, and arms should be parallel to the floor.

Keep elbows at shoulder height as you pull your hands toward the chest.

Straighten arms as you return the starting position.

Repeat up to 10 times.

The patient may hold a light weight in each hand or use an elastic exercise band anchored behind the chair to make the exercise a little harder.

Bring in the band—Sit in a chair or wheelchair.

Feet flat on the floor.

Lift knees one after the other (right, left, right left).

Seated marching.

Each knee lift counts as 1.

Work up to 60 without stopping.

Dance away the night—Sit in a chair or wheelchair.

Begin with knees and feet as close together as possible.

Lift the left knee about ½ inch.

Move the left leg 5–6 inches out to the left side.

Return to starting position.

Repeat up to 10 times.

Repeat the sequence using the right leg.

An ankle weight may be used on the "working" leg to make the exercise a little harder.

Sitting ballet—Sit in a chair or wheelchair.

Feet flat on the floor.

Lift the heels 1–3 inches off the floor.

Keep toes in contact with the floor.

Count to 5.

Lower to starting position.

Repeat up to 10 times.

Up and at 'em—Sit in a chair or locked wheelchair. Have a stable surface in directly in front of the patient for balance and support.

Place hands on the arms of the chair or cross the arms over chest.

Feet flat on the floor.

Lean forward slightly, and push through legs to stand completely upright.

Count to 5.

Slowly return to a seated position using hands for support or crossing arms over chest.

Lying Exercises

Choose at least 2 exercises from each exercise group.

Head turns

Look over the right shoulder; count to 5.

Look over the left shoulder; count to 5.

Repeat the sequence 5 times.

Head tilts

While looking forward, tilt head to the right shoulder; count to 5.

While looking forward, tilt head to the left shoulder; count to 5.

Repeat the sequence 5 times.

"I don't know's"

Look forward and shrug shoulders up to ears; count to 5.

Lower shoulders to starting position; count to 5.

Repeat sequence 5 times.

Shoulder rolls

Look forward; roll both shoulders forward.

Repeat 5 times.

Look forward; roll both shoulders backward.

Repeat 5 times.

Airplanes

Hold arm straight out to the front.

Circle straight arm 5 times to the right and 5 times to the left.

Repeat the sequence using the other arm.

(If able can do both arms at the same time.)

Teapot side bends—Place patient in a semi-upright position.

Place one arm above your head (slightly bent).

Bend sideways at the waist away from the raised arm.

Return to the starting position.

Repeat 5 times to one side then switch arms and repeat sequence to the other side.

Modification for those who cannot successfully reach arm above head:

Place hand on the head to do the side bend.

Clap those hands—Place patient supine or in a semi-upright position.

Hold arms out to sides at shoulder height.

Palms face inward.

Cross right arm over body to touch the left arm or hand.

Count to 5.

Return to starting position.

Repeat up to 10 times.

Switch arms and repeat up to 10 times.

Point those toes—Place patient in a supine or semi-upright position. (A rolled towel or sheet may be placed under knees.)

Keep legs as straight as possible.

Pump feet back and forth (flex and point).

Repeat up to 10 times.

Ankle circles—Place patient in a supine or semi-upright position with a rolled towel or sheet under knees.

Keep legs as straight as possible.

Circle one ankle at a time.

Complete up to 10 circles with each ankle.

(continued)

Table 4.7 *Continued*

Lying Exercises (*cont.*)

Popeye exercise—Place the patient in a semi-upright position.
  Hold right arm straight down at the side.
  Keep elbow glued to the waist.
  Palm facing forward.
  Bend elbow.
  Lift palm up to the shoulder.
  Return to the starting position.
  Repeat up to 10 times with the right arm.
  Switch to the left arm and repeat up to 10 times.
    A weight or elastic exercise band may be used to make the exercise a little more difficult.

Hugs
  Hold slightly bent arms horizontally out to your sides.
  Palms face each other.
  Bring arms in toward the center and give yourself a hug.
  Count to 5.
  Open arms out to the side (keeping them slightly bent).
  Repeat the sequence up to 10 times.
    A weight may be held in each hand to make the exercise a little more difficult.

Wave to the crowd—Place the patient in a semi-upright position.
  Hold arms as straight as possible to the front and below shoulder height.
  Raise the arms to shoulder height or slightly above.
  Count to 5.
  Return to start position.
  Repeat up to 10 times.

Scrub the countertop—Place the patient in a semi-upright position.
  Hold arms as straight as possible out to the front.
  Palms should face down and arms should be parallel to the floor.
  Keep elbows at shoulder height as you pull your hands toward the chest.
  Straighten arms as you return the starting position.
  Repeat up to 10 times.

Bring in the band—Place the patient in a semi-upright position.
  Bend both knees.
  Feet flat on the bed.
  Lift one knee at a time as if marching.
  Repeat right, left, right, left.
  Each lift counts as 1.
  Complete up to 60 lifts.

Dance away the night—Place patient in a supine or semi-upright position.
  Begin with legs as straight as possible and close together.
  Slide the right leg out to the side.
  Count to 5.
  Return to starting position.
  Repeat up to 10 times with each leg.
    Or
  Lift leg 1/4 inch and move out to the side.
  Return to start position.
    Or
  Begin in a side-lying position.
  Lift the top leg upward about 5–10 inches.
  Return to start position.
  Repeat on each leg.

Table 4.8 Recommendations for Walking/Ambulation Groups

Park and Dine
1. Assign a "parking lot" some distance from the main dining room and unit dining rooms
2. Residents who can ambulate leave wheelchairs in the "parking lot" and walk to meals
3. Staff members are available immediately prior to meals to assist residents to walk from the "parking lot" to the dining room for meals
4. Volunteers and families may be helpful and should be encouraged to assist
5. The residents might enjoy the use of one staff member dressed as a "chauffeur" with hat and gloves to make them feel special

Walking Across America (or the World)
1. Encourage residents to participate in walking as a group exercise
2. Assign a special place—city or state—as the goal to reach
3. Use pictures, signs, and posters to encourage excitement and depict the theme of the destination
4. Record the actual miles to arrive
5. Use music or props to help
6. Keep records of the "miles" residents walk
7. Award prizes to the residents who arrive at the destination in the required trip time

Special Walks
1. A walk around the facility outside
2. A walk to a lemonade stand (which has been provided by dining services)
3. A "nature" walk with pictures or articles with a nature theme along the way
4. A scavenger hunt with directions to certain locations to find the prizes
5. "Trick or treat" on Halloween
6. A walk to the "zoo" with zoo animals pictured on the walls along the way
7. Special "music to walk by" (like rock and roll, big band sounds, western swing, jazz, or whatever the residents request)
8. "March" with actual instruments (or activity rhythm instruments)

activities to attain the goal. For individuals residing in long-term care settings, organizational support for restorative care is critical. Caregivers in these facilities must have the education, training, and support to implement restorative activities. Supervision of the caregivers to ensure that activities are being carried out as planned and are being delivered safely is important (see Tables 4.9 & 4.10). Communication among caregivers will ensure consistency and improve the likelihood of attaining desired outcomes. Finally, exercising flexibility and creativity in designing activities to reach restorative goals will improve compliance and outcomes. Restorative caregiving principles can be incorporated into volunteer-run dining (Musson, Frye, & Nash, 1997) and exercise programs (Buettner & Fitzsimmons, 2002; Fitzsimmons, 2001; Palo-Bengtsson & Ekman, 2002), activities with animals (Fick, 1993; Gammonley & Yates, 1991; Kaiser, Spence, McGavin, Struble, Keilman, 2002) and children

Table 4.9 Recommendations for Well-Attended Group Classes

Movin' and Groovin'
1. Find a busy, central location.
2. Play popular or entertaining music with a lively beat.
3. Get the staff who pass by involved, even if only for a few minutes.
4. Use lots of leader energy.
5. Provide props like weights or weight-like devices.
6. Change the themes—provide Mexican music with hats, western music with guns and lassos.

Wheelchair Basketball—"The Hoop Group"
1. A good group for staff interested in sports.
2. Encourage using arms to propel wheelchairs toward the basketball hoops.
3. Toss basketballs.
4. Try dribbling, bouncing, and tossing.
5. Keep score and award prizes.
6. Announce and post the winners.
7. Form teams and give funny names.
8. Get staff to participate by also getting into the wheelchairs to make baskets.

Golf or Croquet or Modified Football—"Clubs, Mallets, and Kicks"
1. For residents who can ambulate.
2. Strengthen arms and legs with practicing swings.
3. Make up fun and therapeutic rules of participation.
4. Get staff to actually compete with residents.
5. Use softballs and plastic clubs, etc.
6. List the teams and team members.
7. Make it fun.

Table 4.10 Group Classes Especially for Those with Cognitive Impairment

Wheelchair Dancing
1. Residents in a wheelchair need to be taught to propel themselves.
2. Use music and assist residents to move wheelchairs with the music.
3. Go "square dancing" or "line dancing."
4. Incorporate the help of residents who ambulate to assist in moving wheelchairs around.
5. Get the help of staff.
6. Make the music fun.

Chair Aerobics
1. Modify an aerobic exercise program for chairbound residents.
2. Use a specified exercise program.
3. Use upbeat music.
4. Do repetitions for muscle building.
5. Use props like sticks, poles, weights, and scarves and incorporate them into the exercises to add variety.

Musical Chairs
1. An adaptation to the children's game where music is played as residents walk around the chairs, then sit down when the music stops.
2. Losers still participate by forming a "loser" line of chairs that grows as the "winners" line decreases; this keeps everyone active.
3. Provide guidance and supervision.
4. Give prizes to the winners.
5. Give recognition to everyone.

Alzheimer's Groups
1. Provide adaptations of exercise programs to accommodate the cognitively impaired resident.
2. Keep them busy and give individual attention.
3. Group the residents according to skill levels so all participate.
4. Music and motion are well received by this group.
5. Build in lots of laughter and fun.
6. Use bells or rhythm instruments that require arm motion.
7. Always recognize safety precautions.

(Hamilton et al., 1999; Krout & Pogorzala, 2002), seasonal and holiday events, gardening and outdoor activities, and offsite trips. For older adults and caregivers, participating in restorative care can be satisfying and rewarding. Achieving independence in performing ADLs restores dignity and self-esteem for the older adult and satisfaction for the caregiver.

REFERENCES

Allen, R., Jackson, S., Marsden, H., McLellan, D.L., & Gore, S. (2002). Transferring people safely with manual handling equipment. *Clinical Rehabilitation, 16*(3), 329–337.

Amella, E.J. (1998). Assessment and management of eating and feeding difficulties for older people: A NICHE protocol. *Geriatric Nursing, 19*(5), 269–275.

Axelrod, S. Mobility. (1999). *Restorative nursing: A training manual for nursing assistants.* C.A. Tracey (Ed.), Glenview, IL: Association of Rehabilitation Nurses.

Barrick, A.L., Rader, J., Hoeffer, B., & Sloane P.D. (2001). *Bathing without a battle.* New York, NY: Springer Publishing Co.

Baum, E.E., Jarjoura, D., Polen, A.E., Faur, D., & Rutecki, G. (2003). Effectiveness of a group exercise program in a long-term care facility: A randomized pilot trial. *Journal of the American Medical Directors Association, 4*(2), 74–80.

Beck C., Heacock, P., Mercer, S.O., Walls, R.C., Rapp, C.G., & Vogelpohl, T.S. (1997). Improving dressing behavior in cognitively impaired nursing home residents. *Nursing Research, 46*(3), 126–131.

Birch, S., & Coggins, T. (2003). No-rinse, one-step bed bath: The effects on the occurrence of skin tears in a long-term care setting. *Ostomy Wound Management, 49*(1), 64–67.

Blair, C.E. (1999). Effect of self-care ADLs on self-esteem of intact nursing home residents. *Issues in Mental Health Nursing, 20*(6), 559–570.

Blaum, C.S., Fries, B.E., & Fiatarone, M.A. (1995). Factors associated with low body mass index and weight loss in nursing home residents. *Journal of Gerontology, 50*(3), M162–M168.

Buettner, L.L., & Fitzsimmons, S. (2002). AD-venture program: therapeutic biking for the treatment of depression in long-term care residents with dementia. *American Journal of Alzheimer Disease and Other Dementias, 17*(2), 121–127.

Burgio, L.D., McCormick, K.A., Scheve, A.S., Engel, B.T., Hawkins, A., & Leahy, E. (1994). The effects of changing prompted voiding schedules in the treatment of incontinence in nursing home residents. *Journal of the American Geriatrics Society, 42*(3), 315–320.

Cole, S.L. (1992). Dress for success: A nurse's knowledge of simple clothing adaptations and dressing aids may make the difference between rehabilitation success and failure. *Geriatric Nursing, 13*(4), 217–221.

Colling, J., Ouslander, J., Hadley, B.J., Eisch, J., & Campbell, E. (1992). The effects of patterned urge-response toileting (PURT) on urinary incontinence among nursing home residents. *Journal of the American Geriatrics Society, 40,* 135–141.

Crogan, N.L, & Shultz, J.A. (2002). Nursing assistants' perceptions of barriers to nutrition care for residents in long-term care facilities. *Journal of Nursing Staff Development, 16*(5), 216–221.

Daynard, D., Yassi, A., Cooper, J.E., Tate, R., Norman, R., & Wells, R. (2001). Biochemical analysis of peak and cumulative spinal loads during simulated patient-handling activities: A subsidy of a randomized controlled trial to prevent lift and transfer injury of health care workers. *Appl Ergon, 32*(3), 199–214.

Elmstahl, S., Blabolil, V., Fex, G., Kuller, R., & Steen, B. (1987). Hospital nutrition in geriatric long-term care medicine. Effects of a changed meal environment. *Comprehensive Gerontology, 1*(1), 29–33.

Engel, B.T., Burgio, L.D., McCormick, K.A., Hawkins, A.M., Scheve, A.S., & Leahy, E. (1990). Behavioral treatment of incontinence in the long-term care setting. *Journal of the American Geriatrics Society, 38,* 361–363.

Engelman, K., Mathews, R., & Altus, D. (2002). Restoring dressing independence in persons with Alzheimer's disease: A pilot study. *American Journal of Alzheimer's Disease and Other Dementias, 17*(1), 37–43.

Evans, W.J. (1995). Effects of exercise on body composition and functional capacity of the elderly. *Journals of Gerontology A: Biological, Medical, Psychological and Social Sciences, 50,* Spec No, 147–150.

Evans, W.J. (1999). Exercise training guidelines for the elderly. *Med Sci Sports Exerc, 31*(1), 12–17.

Fiatarone, M.A., O'Neil, E.F., Ryan, N.D., Clements, K.M., Solares, G.R., Nelson, M.E., Roberts, S.B., Kehayias, J.J., Lipsitz, L.A., & Evans, W.J. (1994). Exercise training and nutritional supplementation for physical frailty in very elderly people. *The New England Journal of Medicine, 330*(25), 1769–1775.

Fick, K.M. (1993). The influence of an animal on social interactions of nursing home residents in a group setting. *American Journal of Occupational Therapy, 47*(6), 529–534.

Fitzsimmons, S. (2001). Easy rider wheelchair biking. A nursing-recreation therapy clinical trial for the treatment of depression. *Journal of Gerontological Nursing, 27*(5), 14–23.

Galinsky, T., Waters, T., & Malit, B. (2001). Overexertion injuries in home health care workers and the need for ergonomics. *Home Health Care Services Quarterly, 20*(3), 57–73.

Gammonley, J., & Yates, J. (1991). Pet projects: Animal assisted therapy in nursing homes. *Journal of Gerontological Nursing, 17*(1), 12–15.

Garg, A., Owen, B., Beller, D., & Banaag, J. (1991). A biomechanical and ergonomic evaluation of patient transferring tasks: Bed to wheelchair and wheelchair to bed. *Ergonomics, 34*(3), 289–312.

Garg, A., Owen, B.D., & Carlson, B. (1992). An ergonomic evaluation of nursing assistants' job in a nursing home. *Ergonomics, 35*(9), 979–995.

Glenn, J. (2003). Restorative nursing bladder training program: Recommending a strategy. *Rehabilitation Nursing, 28*(1), 15–22.

Hagen, B., Armstrong-Esther, C., & Sandilands, M. (2003). On a happier note: Validation of musical exercise for older persons in long-term care settings. *International Journal of Nursing Studies, 40*(4), 347–357.

Hamilton, G., Brown, S., Alonzo, T., Glover, M., Mersereau, Y., & Willson, P. (1999). Building community for the long-term: an intergenerational commitment. *Gerontologist, 39*(2), 235–238.

Heacock, P.R., Beck, C.M., Souder, E., & Mercer, S. (1997). Assessing dressing ability in dementia. *Geriatric Nursing, 18*(3), 107–111.

Hoeffer, B., Rader, J., McKenzie, D., Lavelle, M., & Stewart, B. (1997). Reducing aggressive behavior during bathing cognitively nursing home residents. *Journal of Gerontological Nursing, 23*(5), 16–23.

Hu, T., Igou, J.F., Kaltreider, L., Yu, L.C., Rohmer, T.J., Dennis, P.J., Craighead, W.E., Hadley, E.C., & Ory, M.G. (1989). A clinical trial of a behavioral therapy to reduce urinary incontinence in nursing homes. Outcome and implications. *Journal of the American Medical Association, 262*(18), 2538–2539.

Kaiser, L., Spence, L.J., McGavin, L., Struble, L., & Keilman, L. (2002). A dog and a "happy person" visit nursing home residents. *Western Journal of Nursing Research, 24*(6), 671–683.

Kayser-Jones, J. (1996). Mealtime in nursing homes: The importance of individualized care. *Journal of Gerontological Nursing, 22*(3), 26–31.

Kayser-Jones, J. (1997). Inadequate staffing at mealtime: Implications for nursing and health policy. *Journal of Gerontological Nursing, 23*, 14–21.

Kayser-Jones, J., & Schell, E. (1997a). The effect of staffing on the quality of care at mealtime. *Nursing Outlook, 45*, 64–72.

Kayser-Jones, J., & Schell, E. (1997b). The mealtime experience of a cognitively impaired elder. Ineffective and effective strategies. *Journal of Gerontological Nursing, 23*, 33–37.

Koroknay, V.J., Werner, P., Cohen-Mansfield, J., & Braun, J.V. (1995). Maintaining ambulation in the frail nursing home resident: A nursing administered walking program. *Journal of Gerontological Nursing, 21*(11), 18–24.

Kovach, C.R., & Meyer-Arnold, E.A. (1997). Preventing agitated behaviors during bath time. *Geriatric Nursing, 18*(3), 112–114.

Kraker, K., & Vajdik, C. (1997). Designating the environment to make bathing pleasant in nursing homes. *Journal of Gerontological Nursing, 23*(5), 50–51.

Krout, J.A., & Pogorzala, C.H. (2002). An intergenerational partnership between a college and congregate housing facility: How it works, what it means. *Gerontologist, 42*(6), 853–858.

Lange-Alberts, M., & Shott, S. (1994). Nutritional intake: Use of touch and verbal cueing. *Journal of Gerontological Nursing, 20*, 36–40.

Lazowski, D.A., Ecclestone, N.A., Myers, A.M., Paterson, D.H., Tudor-Locke, C., Fitzgerald, C., Jones, G., Shima, N., & Cunningham, D.A. (1999). A randomized outcome evaluation of group exercise programs in long-term care institutions. *Journals of Gerontology A: Biological, Medical, Psychological and Social Sciences, 54*(12), M621–M628.

Lekan-Rutledge, D. (2000). Diffusion of innovation a model for implementation of prompted voiding in long-term care settings. *Journal of Gerontological Nursing, 26*(4), 25–33.

Li, F., Harmer, P., McAuley, E., Fisher, K.J., Duncan, T.E., & Duncan, S.C. (2001). Tai chi, self-efficacy, and physical function in the elderly. *Preventive Science, 2*(4), 229–39.

Lim, Y.M. (2003). Nursing intervention for grooming of elders with mild cognitive impairments in Korea. *Geriatric Nursing, 24*(1), 11–15.

Lord, S.R., & Bashford, G.M. (1996). Shoe characteristics and balance in older women. *Journal of the American Geriatrics Society, 44*, 429–433.

Lynch, R.M., & Freund, A. (2000). Short-term efficacy of back injury intervention project for patient care providers at one hospital. *AIHAJ, 61*(2), 290–294.

MacRae, P.G., Asplund, L.A., Schnelle, J.F., Ouslander, J.G., Abrahamse, A., & Morris, C. (1996). A walking program for nursing home residents: Effects on walk endurance, physical activity, mobility, and quality of life. *Journal of the American Geriatrics Society, 44*(2), 175–180.

Martin, L.S. (1998). Developing a C.R.A.F.T. approach to resident bathing. *Canadian Nursing Home, 9*(2), 5–8.

Mathews, R.M., Clair, A.A., & Kosloski, K. (2001). Keeping the beat: Use of rhythmic music during exercise activities for the elderly with dementia. *American Journal of Alzheimer Disease and Other Dementia, 16*(6), 377–380.

Mathey, M.F., Siebelink, E., de Graaf, C., & Van Staveren, W.A. (2001). Flavor enhancement of food improves dietary intake and nutritional status of elderly nursing home residents. *Journal of Gerontology, 56*(4), M200–M2005.

Mathey, M.F., Vanneste, V.G., de Graaf, C., de Groot, L.C., & van Staveren, W.A. (2001). Health effect of improved meal ambiance in a Dutch nursing home: A 1-year intervention study. *Preventive Medicine, 32*(5), 416–423.

Maxfield, M.C., Lewis, R.E., & Cannon, S. (1996). Training staff to prevent aggressive behavior of cognitively impaired elderly patients during bathing and grooming. *Journal of Gerontological Nursing, 22*(1), 37–43.

Miller, M.F. (1997). Physically aggressive resident behavior during hygienic care. *Journal of Gerontological Nursing, 23*(5), 24–39.

Morley, J.E., & Kraenzle, D. (1994). Causes of weight loss in a community nursing home. *Journal of the American Geriatrics Society, 42*(6), 583–585.

Morley, J.E., & Silver, A.J. (1995). Nutritional issues in nursing home care. *Annals of Internal Medicine, 1*(11), 850–859.

Morris, J.N., Fiaterone, M., Kiely, D.K., Belleville-Taylor, P., Murphy, K., Littlehale, S., Ooi, W.L., O'Neill, E., & Doyle, N. (1999). Nursing rehabilitation and exercise strategies in the nursing home. *Journals of Gerontology A: Biological, Medical, Psychological and Social Sciences, 54*(10), M494–M500.

Mulrow, C.D., Gerety, M.B., Kanten, D., Cornell, J.E., DeNino, L.A., Chiodo, L., Aguilar, C., O'Neil, M.B., Rosenberg, J., & Solis, R.M. (1994). A randomized trial of physical rehabilitation for very frail nursing home residents. *Journal of the American Medical Association, 271*(7), 519–524.

Musson, N.D., Frye, G.D., & Nash, M. (1997). Silver spoons: Supervised volunteers provide feeding of patients. *Geriatric Nursing, 17,* 18–19.

Nelson, A., Lloyd., J.D., Menzel, N., & Gross., C. (2003). Preventing nursing back injuries: Redesigning patient handling tasks. *American Association of Occupational Health Nursing, 51*(3), 126–34.

Nowalk, M.P., Predergast, J.M., Bayles, C.M., D'Amico, F.J., & Colvin, G.C. (2001). A randomized trial of exercise programs among older individuals living in long-term care facilities: The FallsFREE program. *Journal of American Geriatrics Society, 49*(7), 859–865.

Osborn, C., & Marshall, M. (1993). Self-feeding performance in nursing home residents. *Journal of Gerontological Nursing, 19,* 7–14.

Owen, B.D., Keene, K., & Olson, S. (2002). An ergonomic approach to reducing back/shoulder stress in hospital nursing personnel: A five year follow up. *International Journal of Nursing Studies, 39*(3), 295–302.

Palo-Bengtsson, L., & Ekman, S.L. (2002). Emotional response to social dancing and walks in persons with dementia. *American Journal of Alzheimer Disease and Other Dementias, 17*(3), 149–153.

Pawlson, L.G., Goodwin, M., & Keith, K. (1986). Wheelchair use by ambulatory nursing home residents. *Journal of the American Geriatrics Society, 34*(12), 860–864.

Przybylski, B.R., Dumont, E.D., Watkins, M.E., Warren, S.A., Beaulne, A.P., & Lier, D.A. (1996). Outcomes of enhanced physical and occupational therapy service in a nursing home setting. *Archives of Physical Medicine and Rehabilitation, 77*(6), 554–561.

Pyle, M.A., Massie, M., & Nelson, S. (1998). A pilot study on improving oral care in long-term care settings—Part I—Oral health assessment and II—Procedures and outcomes. *Journal of Gerontological Nursing, 24*(10), 31–38.

Rader, J., Lavelle, M., Hoeffer, B., & McKenzie, D. (1996). Maintaining cleanliness: An individualized approach. *Journal of Gerontological Nursing, 22*(3), 32–38.

Ragneskog, H., Brane, G., Karlsson, I., & Kihlgren, M. (1996). Influence of dinner music on food intake and symptoms common in dementia. *Scandinavian Journal of Caring Sciences, 10*(1), 11–17.

Ragneskog, H., Kihlgren, M., Karlsson, I., & Norberg, A. (1996). Dinner music for demented patients: analysis of video-recorded observations. *Clinical Nursing Research, 5*(3), 262–277.

Remsburg, R.E. (1999b). Activities of daily living. In C.A. Tracey (Ed.), *Restorative nursing: A training manual for nursing assistants.* Glenview, IL: Association of Rehabilitation Nurses.

Remsburg, R.E. (1999b). The NA's role in restorative care. In C.A. Tracey (Ed.), *Restorative nursing: A training manual for nursing assistants.* Glenview, IL: Association of Rehabilitation Nurses.

Remsburg, R.E., Armacost, K.A., Radu, C., & Bennett, R.G. (1999). Two models of restorative care in the nursing home: Designated versus integrated restorative nursing assistants. *Geriatric Nursing, 20*(6), 321–326.

Remsburg, R.E., Armacost, K.A., Radu, C., & Bennett, R.G. (2001). Impact of a restorative care program in the nursing home. *Educational Gerontology, 27,* 261–280.

Remsburg, R.E., Luking, A., Baran, P., Radu, C., Pineda, D., Bennett, R.G., & Tayback, M. (2001). Impact of a buffet-style dining program on weight and biochemical indicators of nutritional status in nursing home residents: A pilot study. *Journal of the American Dietetic Association, 101*(12), 1460–1463.

Robbins, S., Gouw, G.J., & McClaran, J. (1992). Shoe sole thickness and hardness influence balance in older men. *Journal of the American Geriatrics Society, 40,* 1089–1094.

Rogers, J.C., Holm, M.B., Burgio, L.D., Granieri, E., Hsu, C., Hardin, J.M., & McDowell, B.J. (1999). Improving morning care routines of nursing home residents with dementia. *Journal of the American Geriatrics Society, 47*(9), 1049–1057.

Schnelle, J.F. (1990). Treatment of urinary incontinence in nursing home patients by prompted voiding. *Journal of the American Geriatrics Society, 38,* 356–360.

Schnelle, J.F, Alessi, C., Simmons, S.F., Al-Samarrai, N.R., Beck, J.G., & Ouslander, J.G. (2002). Translating clinical research into practice: A randomized controlled trial of exercise and incontinence care with nursing home residents. *Journal of the American Geriatrics Society, 50*(9), 1476–1483.

Schnelle, J.F, Kapur, K., Alessi, C., Osterweil, D., Beck, J.G., Al-Samarrai, N.R., & Ouslander, J.G. (2003). Does an exercise and incontinence intervention save healthcare costs in a nursing home population? *Journal of the American Geriatrics Society, 51*(2), 161–168.

Schnelle, J.F., MacRae, P.G., Ouslander, J.G., Simmons, S.F., & Nitta, M. (1995). Functional incidental training, mobility performance, and incontinence care with nursing home residents. *Journal of American Geriatrics Society, 43*(12), 1356–1362.

Schnelle, J.F., Newman, D., White, M., Abbey, J., Wallston, K.A., Fogarty, T., & Ory, M. (1993). Maintaining continence in nursing home residents through application of industrial quality control. *Gerontologist, 33,* 114–121.

Shatenstein, B., Ska, B., & Ferland, G. (2001). Employee reactions to the introduction of a bulk food distribution system in a nursing home. *Canadian Journal of Dietary Practice and Research, 62*(1), 18–25.

Simmons, S.F., Alessi, C., & Schnelle, J.F. (2001). An intervention to increase fluid intake in nursing home residents: Prompting and preference compliance. *Journal of the American Geriatrics Society, 49*(7), 926–933.

Simmons, S.F., Babineau, S., Garcia, E., & Schnelle, J.F. (2002). Quality assessment in nursing homes by systematic direct observation: Feeding assistance. *Journal of Gerontology, 57*(10), M665–M671.

Simmons, S.F., Osterweil, D., & Schnelle, J.F. (2001). Improving food intake in nursing home residents with feeding assistance: A staffing analysis. *J Gerontol A Biol Sci Med Sci, 56*(12), M790–M794.

Simmons, S.F., Schnelle, J.F., MacRae, P.G., & Ouslander, J.G. (1995). Wheelchairs as mobility restraints: Predictors of wheelchair activity in nonambulatory nursing home residents. *Journal of the American Geriatrics Society, 43*(4), 384–388.

Skewes, S.M. (1997). Bathing: It's a tough job! *Journal of Gerontological Nursing, 23*(5), 45–49.

Sloane, P.D., Rader, J., Barrick, A.L., Hoeffer, B., Dwyer, S., McKenzie, D., Lavelle, M., Buckwalter, K., Arring-ton, L., & Pruitt, T. (1995). Bathing persons with dementia. *The Gerontologist, 35*(5), 672–678.

Smith, D.B. (1998). The culture of long-term care: Impact on a continence care program. *Urology Nursing, 18*(4), 291–295.

Steele, C.M., Greenwood, C., Ens, I., Robertson, C., & Seidman-Carlson, R. (1997). Mealtime difficulties in a home for the aged: Not just dysphagia. *Dysphagia, 12*(1), 43–50.

Taggart, H.M. (2002). Effects of Tai chi exercise on balance, functional mobility, and fear of falling among older women. *Applied Nursing Research, 15*(4), 235–242.

Tappen, R.M. (1994). The effect of skill training on functional abilities of nursing home residents with dementia. *Research in Nursing and Health, 17,* 159–165.

Tappen, R.M., Roach, K.E., Applegate, E.B., & Stowell, P. (2000). Effect of a combined walking and conversation intervention on functional mobility of nursing home residents with Alzheimer disease. *Alzheimer Disease and Associated Disorders, 14*(4), 196–201.

Van Ort, S., & Phillips, L. (1995). Nursing interventions to promote functional feeding. *Journal of Gerontological Nursing, 21,* 6–14.

Wu, G. (2002). Evaluation of the effectiveness of Tai chi for improving balance and preventing falls in the older population—A review. *Journal of the American Geriatrics Society, 50*(4), 746–754.

Yassi, A., Cooper, J.E., Tate, R.B., Gerlach, S., Muir, M., Trottier, J., & Massey, K. (2001). A randomized controlled trial to prevent patient lift and transfer injuries of health care workers. *Spine, 26*(16), 1739–1746.

Zhuang, Z., Stobbe, T.J., Collins, J.W., Hsiao, H., & Hobbs, G.R. (1999). Biomechanical evaluation of assistive devices for transferring residents. *Applied Ergonomics, 30*(4), 285–924.

Zhuang, Z., Stobbe, T.J., Collins, J.W., Hsiao, H., & Hobbs, G.R. (2000). Psychophysical assessment of assistive devices for transferring patients/residents. *Applied Ergonomics, 31*(1), 35–44.

CHAPTER 5

Motivating the Older Adult to Engage in Restorative Care

Barbara Resnick

Health care providers working with older adults may know about restorative care, have the skills to engage in this type of caregiving, and believe in the many benefits of engaging in restorative care activities. Unfortunately, older individuals may not be willing to participate in restorative care activities. It is not unusual for older adults in any setting to decide that they need to be cared for with regard to personal care activities. These individuals may be highly motivated to get the care-providing services they believe they need, whether from families or paid caregivers. Consequently, a major aspect of implementing a restorative care program is motivating the older adult to engage in these activities.

Motivation is an important factor in the older adult's ability to recover from a disabling event and perform functional activities (Bootsma-van der Wiel et al., 2001; Kemp, 1988; Resnick, 1996). Unfortunately, motivation is not often addressed, nor are interventions utilized to improve motivation with regard to performance of functional activities. Rather, the older adult is perceived as unwilling to participate, and care providers perform the necessary functional act by bathing, and/or dressing the older adult and using a wheelchair for mobility rather than encouraging ambulation (Waters, 1994). This process results in a further decline in function.

Motivation comes from within the individual and refers to the need, drive, or desire to act in a certain way to achieve a certain end. Motivation is behavior specific and must be considered for any activity. The Wheel of Motivation (Figure 5.1) is a useful model to consider all the potential factors that can influence motivation

to perform a specific activity (Resnick, 1996; 1998; 1999a and b). Descriptions of the most relevant factors are provided in Table 5.1, as are specific interventions that can be used to help strengthen motivation.

Health care providers working with older adults can have a significant influence on motivation by strengthening older adults' beliefs about their abilities to perform a given activity, and their beliefs about the benefits of that activity. In addition, individualized care that includes verbal encouragement to perform an activity, expressed in a kind and caring way, lets these individuals know that the care provider is invested in them and cares enough to spend time and energy in getting them to perform functional activities. Flexibility with regard to individual differences and desires, for example, setting up a bathing or eating schedule that may not conform to traditional caregiving times (i.e., changing set mealtimes or bathing times) can also help to motivate these individuals to perform the behavior.

Identification of goals, both short and long term, has been reported to influence motivation to perform functional activities in older adults (Resnick, 1998a; 1999a). In some cases the goals were specific, such as being able to walk across the room or get up from a chair. Other individuals reported more general goals such as maintaining independence, maintaining a certain routine, or maintaining their pride and modesty during bathing and dressing activities. Nurses should work with older adults to help them identify goals that are clear, specific, and attainable. The goals should be moderately difficult, and ideally they should come from the individual. Older adults with cognitive im-

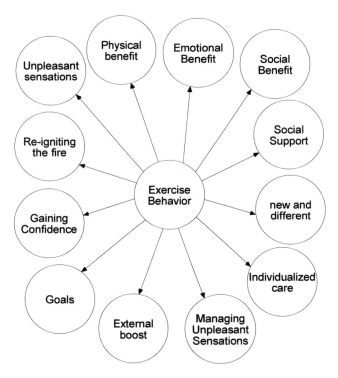

FIGURE 5.1 The Wheel of Motivation.

TABLE 5.1 Components of the Wheel of Motivation and Specific Interventions to Improve Motivation

Wheel Components	Specific Interventions to Improve Motivation to Perform Functional Activities
Beliefs	1. Verbally encourage older adult about capability to perform and the benefits of performance.
	2. Expose older adult to role models (similar others who successfully perform the activity).
	3. Decrease unpleasant sensations associated with the activity.
	4. Encourage actual performance/practice of the activity.
Unpleasant physical sensations (pain, fear)	1. Facilitate appropriate use of pain medications to relieve discomfort.
	2. Use alternative measures such as heat/ice to relieve pain associated with the activity.
	3. Cognitive therapy:
	• Explore thoughts and feelings related to sensations.
	• Help patient develop a more realistic attitude about the pain (e.g., pain will not cause further bone damage).
	• Use relaxation and distraction techniques.
	• Use graded exposure to overcome fear of falling.
Individualized care	1. Demonstrate kindness and caring to the patient.
	2. Use humor.
	3. Use positive reinforcement following a desired behavior.
	4. Recognize individual needs and differences, such as by setting a rest period or providing a favorite snack.
Spirituality	1. Explore the influence of spirituality and traditional religion and, as appropriate, encourage the patient to participate in this.
	2. Physically being with the older adult, and listening.
	3. Use life review.
	4. Encourage spiritual experiences—pets, children, journal keeping, reading, friends, prayer.
Social support	1. Evaluate the presence and adequacy of social network.
	2. Teach significant other(s) to verbally encourage/reinforce the desired behavior.
	3. Use social supports as a source of goal identification.
Self-determination	1. Recognize underlying personality, and build interventions to improve motivation based on that personality.
Goal identification	1. Develop appropriate realistic goals with the older adult.
	2. Set goals that can be met in a short time—a day, a week.
	3. Set goals that are challenging but attainable.
	4. Set goals that are clear and specific.

pairment can identify simple goals (e.g., walking to the dining room) that, if repeated frequently, can help sustain motivation to perform the desired activity. Family and friends provide an excellent source of goals. Older adults can be encouraged to get up and dress so they can go out to lunch with a friend, or to exercise daily to maintain their strength and function and be able to go to a daughter's home for a visit.

It is particularly important to explore with each older adult any unpleasant sensations experienced during the activity of interest. If there is pain or fear of falling associated with bathing, dressing, or walking, the desired functional activity will not likely be performed. These unpleasant sensations must be decreased or eliminated if the behavior is to occur. Sometimes simply explaining to the older adult that these are normal sensations associated with a given activity or giving pain medication prior to the activity can help the individual cope with the unpleasant sensations.

NORMAL AGE CHANGES IN MOTIVATION

Motivation changes with age and is different than it is among younger individuals. These changes, listed in

Table 5.2, include a tendency to be less concerned about major achievements and more interested in tasks that are relevant and meaningful to their daily lives. Older adults do not function well when stressed or rushed, they tend to see a task as being difficult, and they tend to become easily discouraged. This feeling of discouragement results in an unwillingness even to try to perform a task or engage in an activity. Likewise there is a tendency to reset their goals to a lower level. That is when an older women who was functionally independent has a hip fracture, for example, she may not expect to return to her baseline function. Rather she will set a goal that is lower such as ambulating with walker, and not being able to go up and down stairs.

Many normal age changes also have an impact on motivation. The changes most commonly noted involve vision, hearing, sensation, taste, touch, as well as changes in specific body systems (Table 5.3). Sensory changes, such as in the ability to see and hear, can affect motivation or the health care provider's perception of the individual's motivation. With regard to sensory changes, the threshold needed for each sensory modality to be stimulated increases with age, and activation of the corresponding receptors requires stimuli of increased intensity. Therefore, a greater stimulus is needed for the sensation to occur. It is also generally more difficult for older adults to differentiate between different stimuli. If the older adult cannot see or hear the provider and does not perform the requested task,

TABLE 5.2 Age Changes Related to Motivation

1. A shift from achievement motivation to conservative motivation (Older adults want concrete and immediate outcomes that are related to activities of daily living.)
2. A tendency to see a task as being difficult
3. A tendency to feel easily discouraged and a tendency not to initiate behavior as readily
4. Increased difficulty identifying rewards (It helps to use previously used systems. For example, for achievement oriented individuals, it may help to keep track of how often or how much of a desired task is done.)
5. Increased importance of the meaning of a task (They need to see/understand the outcome.)
6. A tendency to do less well on tasks when they are under pressure
7. A tendency to lower their expectations with regard to outcomes
8. Increased importance of the cost of performing a task (The costs commonly associated with exercise include pain, fatigue, and fear of falling.)

TABLE 5.3 Normal Physiological Changes Associated With Aging

System	Age-Associated Changes
Skin	Decreased flexibility due to decreased collagen Increased wrinkles Increased dryness Decreased turgor
Lungs	Decreased compliance due to changes in collagen Decreased FEV1 Decreased total lung volume
Brain	Changes in vascular system, neurons, glial cells Hypoperfusion Atrophy
Heart/Vascular	Decreased response to beta-adrenergic stimulation Decreased cardiac output Decreased cardiac index Decreased compliance of ventricles/arteries Calcification of valves Increased systolic hypertension
Kidney	Decreased ability to concentrate urine, resulting in loss of free water and increased sensitivity to salt Decreased GFR Decreased blood flow
Stomach	Decreased digestive secretion enzymes Increased gastric pH Decreased absorptive surface Decreased motility Decreased blood flow
Immune system	Decreased memory of previous antigenic stimuli Decreased responsiveness to immunization Increased anergy Decreased T cell proliferation and function

the provider may perceive this as lack of motivation. Health care providers must anticipate these normal age changes and alter the environment and clinical interactions to best compensate for losses.

Visual Changes

Age-related changes in vision include decreases in visual acuity, visual fields, dark adaptation, and depth perception, and an elevation in the minimal threshold of light perception. Due to the loss of lens elasticity, there is decreased visual accommodation, resulting in farsightedness. Decreased color discrimination is due to the yellowing of the lens, and decreased ability to see short wavelength colors results in blues and greens being more difficult to see. There is increased sensitivity to glare, making it difficult for older adults to perform an activity when looking into the sunlight. Interventions to help maximize vision in older adults are shown in Table 5.4.

Hearing Changes

A decrease in hearing is also very common in older adults, and approximately 30–50% of those over age 65 have significant hearing loss. Three types of hearing disorders are common in the older population: (1) Presbycusis is the progressive, irreversible bilateral loss of high-tone perception often associated with aging; (2) central deafness results from nerve damage within the brain; and (3) conduction deafness results from blockage or impairment of the mechanical movement in the outer or middle ear. Hearing loss in the elderly is often a combined problem. The majority of the loss is due to auditory nerve changes or deterioration of the structures of the ear. There may also be nerve damage beyond the ear. Presbycusis and central deafness can result in permanent hearing loss. Conduction deafness is reversible. Hearing loss normally progresses from high-tone or high-frequency loss to a general loss of both high and low tones. Consonants, which are higher pitched sounds, are not heard as well. There is decreased speech discrimination, especially when there is background noise. Therefore, providers should remember that giving instructions for an activity while the television or radio is on is not likely to result in a successful translation of information.

Certain cues can indicate that older adults are having trouble hearing. They may increase the volume of their own speech, may not respond to a loud noise, or may turn their head to hear better. Other cues are requests to repeat a statement or inappropriate answers

TABLE 5.4 Interventions to Improve Vision

Make sure objects are in the individual's visual field.
Use large lettering and a contrast in colors (black on white).
Allow the individual time to focus and adjust to the environment.
Avoid glare.
Use night lights to help with dark adaptation problems.
Use the colors red and yellow to stimulate vision.
Mark the edges of stairs and curbs to help with depth perception.

TABLE 5.5 Interventions to Augment Hearing

Ensure that hearing aids are in place and working optimally.
Face the person directly so he or she can lip read.
Use gestures and objects to help with verbal communication.
Touch the person to get his or her attention before speaking.
Speak into the individual's good ear.
DON'T SHOUT. Shouting increases the pitch of the voice, and the elderly do not hear high tones well.
Speak slowly and clearly.
Use amplifiers on telephones and alarms.
Allow the person more time to answer your questions.

from someone who has the cognitive ability to answer correctly. If appropriate, make sure that the individual is using assistive devices to augment hearing, and that these are working correctly. Table 5.5 reviews additional interventions to improve older adults' ability to hear.

Changes in Kinesthetic Sense

Kinesthetic sense helps people to know where their body is in space. With age the receptors in the joints and muscles, which facilitate spatial perception, lose the ability to function. Therefore, balance changes. Older adults walk with a shorter step length, less leg lift, and a wider base, and they have a tendency to lean forward. Consequently, they are less able to stop a fall from occurring. Older adult may have an alteration in posture, may forward and grab onto furniture or assistive devices during transfers and when ambulating, and may complain of dizziness. Interventions to help with changes in kinesthetic sense include placing items within reach of the older individual, giving him or her more time to move, and stressing that exercise will help to improve balance by strengthening muscles.

IMPACT OF CHRONIC ILLNESS ON MOTIVATION

Chronic illnesses are common in older adults and can influence motivation because they influence perceptions of ability (i.e., self-efficacy expectations), long-range outcome expectations, and mood, and may cause pain, fatigue, or shortness of breath, all of which directly impact motivation (Resnick & Spellbring,

2000). The most prevalent chronic illnesses in older adults include arthritis (58% incidence), hearing impairments (36% incidence), hypertension (39% incidence), heart conditions (33% incidence), cataracts (28% incidence), and orthopedic impairments (21% incidence) (The Senior Care Source: Facts, Figures & Forecasts, 2003) .

Unfortunately, it is often difficult to differentiate between chronic disorders and acute illnesses among older adults because many of these problems are intricately intertwined. Acute disorders have chronic sequelae, and many chronic conditions can have acute episodes. Older adults with an acute illness may present with (1) atypical complaints or findings, (2) nonspecific or masked signs and symptoms, (3) symptoms that are confounded by coexisting chronic diseases and age-related changes, or (4) no symptoms at all. The most common atypical presentation of acute illness in the older adult is a change in cognitive function. Subtle changes may be noted in memory, perception, communication, orientation, calculation, comprehension, problem solving, thought processes, language, construction abilities, abstraction, or attention.

Even more directly relevant to restorative care activities is the very common presentation of acute illness in the older adult—a change in functional status. Older individuals may suddenly demonstrate a change in their ability to perform activities of daily living such as eating, bathing, dressing, transferring, toileting, or ambulation. These changes may also occur over the course of several days. Behavior changes can also occur as the presenting sign of an acute illness. There may be episodes of agitation, defined as increased vocal or motor behavior that is disruptive, unsafe, or interferes with personal care activities. Conversely, an individual who is normally active (or normally agitated) may exhibit lethargy and apathy. It is important to consider these changes as acute medical problems before assuming that the individual is simply not motivated or is unable to participate in care-related activities.

IMPACT OF MEDICATIONS ON MOTIVATION

Medications, and the subsequent side effects of medications, have been noted to influence motivation.

Drugs that result in orthostatic hypotension, for example, may make individuals feel dizzy and, consequently, unwilling to stand, transfer, or ambulate. Sensing a feeling of imbalance, these individuals may wisely be concerned about falling and getting hurt and may refuse to transfer or ambulate.

Orthostatic hypotension is defined as a decrease of at least 20 mm Hg in systolic blood pressure when an individual moves from a supine position to a standing position. Homeostatic control of blood pressure and heart rate requires frequent and rapid cardiovascular adjustments as an individual changes from supine to sitting and standing positions throughout the day. Without these adjustments, orthostatic hypotension occurs. Some patients with severe orthostatic hypotension are severely incapacitated, and their caregivers assume a significant burden in their care.

The diagnosis of orthostatic hypotension requires the occurrence of a sustained postural decrease in blood pressure, which may be accompanied by symptoms of cerebral hypoperfusion. While the degree of hypotension required to produce symptoms varies, a decrease of 20 mm Hg or more in systolic blood pressure is one commonly used diagnostic criterion. If blood pressure is assessed for less than 2 minutes following a postural change, the degree of hypotension may be overstated. This is particularly true in, older adults because blunted baroreceptor reflexes are common in otherwise normal individuals.

Treatment for orthostatic hypotension is usually not required in the absence of symptoms. Symptoms of cerebral hypoperfusion include dimming or loss of vision, lightheadedness, dizziness, diaphoresis, diminished hearing, pallor, nausea, and weakness. Severe orthostatic decreases in cerebral perfusion can cause syncope. A comprehensive evaluation of medications and coexisting medical conditions is useful, along with a neurologic examination to search for treatable factors that may be contributing to orthostatic hypotension. Medications that commonly cause orthostatic hypotension include diuretics; cardiovascular medications, particularly those that cause vasodilation; and some antidepressants (particularly the tricyclic antidepressants but can also occur with selective serotonin reuptake inhibitors). Anticipating potential side effects of these medications and monitoring older adult status for them is integral to augmenting motivation. Lying and standing blood pressures should be checked routinely in these individuals during follow up with a primary care provider in the outpatient setting or as part of routine vital signs in institutional settings. Generally, the treatment for orthostatic hypotension is to eliminate the cause (i.e., the medication) if possible and to focus on improving the individual's symptoms rather than on achieving arbitrary blood pressure goals.

IMPACT OF MOOD ON MOTIVATION

Mood, particularly the presence of depression, has likewise been associated with motivation and willingness to engage in functional activities (Jette et al., 1998; Resnick, 1998; 1999a and b). Depression was found to be significantly related to participation in aerobic exercise activity (Rejeski & Brawley, 1997) and to adhering to a home-based exercise program for healthy community-dwelling older adults (Jette et al., 1998). Depression seems to impact motivation indirectly through self-efficacy and outcome expectations (Resnick, 1999). From a motivational perspective, therefore, it is essential to identify and treat depression among older individuals.

Older adults' mood and attitude toward a situation can affect their ability to deal with that situation. When feeling sad and blue, individuals may not have the energy to engage in any activity, particularly new activities or challenges. Depressed individuals may feel the activity is too difficult, and they will not try it. A belief that nothing can be done or attempted results in nothing being attempted and no progress being made. This confirms the individual's feeling of hopelessness. Health care providers may continue to encourage the individual to perform restorative care activities, and the he or she may feel increasingly demoralized.

Certainly, attitude affects feelings, feelings affect what the older adult will do or not do, and in a vicious circle lack of action itself affects attitude, feelings, and motivation. If the older adult believes that he or she cannot do the task at hand, he or she may feel hopeless and low, give up, and do even less, thus further confirming feelings of hopelessness.

Interventions to stop this cycle should be implemented. First it may be helpful to get the older individual to acknowledge these feelings. Even older adults with cognitive impairment can describe feelings they are currently experiencing if caregivers listen to them

and prompt them. Caregivers may need to anticipate these thoughts and feelings and directly ask about them. For example, individuals may experience anxiety, sadness, or despair when asked to perform a specific task. Ask the individuals if they were thinking that they could not cope with the task, could not do it, would never achieve the goal, or would not be able to perform the currently requested task. It is not unusual for older adults to feel that they will never get better, that there is no hope (hopelessness), that walking only makes them feel worse and so maybe they shouldn't walk anymore (fear, worry, confusion), or that their system must be permanently damaged and there is nothing they can do about it (despair, resignation). These kinds of thoughts can result in feelings of useless and failure and a worsening of depression.

Treatment should focus on attempting to help the older individual think more positively. Attempt to help them see what they can do instead of what they can't. Discuss with the individual the worst-case scenario for participating in the activity or for not participating. How might the situation turn out if the older individual does the task at hand, and how will it turn out if he or she does nothing. This discussion provides the nurse, nursing assistant, or other caregiver with an opportunity to review the benefits of restorative care activities in terms of maintaining and improving function and overall health status.

Depression Among Older Adults With Cognitive Disorders

Older adults with Alzheimer's disease tend to have more depressive symptoms, with a higher percentage of these symptoms being related to motivation (Berger, Fratiglioni & Forsell, et al., 1999). Symptoms of mood-related disturbance in older adults include dysphoria, appetite disturbance, feelings of guilt, and thoughts of death or suicidal ideation. Symptoms of motivation-related disturbance include lack of interest, psychomotor change, loss of energy, and concentration difficulties. In Alzheimer's disease, mood-related symptoms are more prevalent in mild to moderate stages, while motivation-related symptoms dominate in moderate to severe stages of the disease. Older adults with a known history of Alzheimer's therefore should be carefully assessed for alterations of mood and motivation, and behavioral treatment should be initiated as indicated, along with medication as indicated by the older adult's primary care provider. The team approach to managing depression and subsequent motivation problems is particularly important because the assessment requires input from all members of the team and treatment may require a combination of drug and behavioral interventions that need to be consistently planned and evaluated.

ADDITIONAL FACTORS THAT INFLUENCE MOTIVATION AMONG OLDER ADULTS

Many additional factors contribute to older adults' motivation to engage in functional activities or exercise. These factors are depicted in Figure 5.1, The Wheel of Motivation. Older adults often say that their basic personality or their so-called lack of motivation or laziness influences their willingness to engage in functional activities (Mulrow et al., 1996; Resnick, 1996; 1998; 2000). It is not unusual for older adults to describe themselves as lazy, particularly when it comes to physical activity and personal care activities. Social issues and cultural expectations (Aller & Coeling, 1995; MacRae et al., 1996), particularly in the institutional setting, influence motivation. As previously stated, if older adults believe they are in the long-term care setting to be "cared for," it is unlikely they will be willing to engage in personal care activities. Increasingly, environmental factors (Saelens, Sallis & Frank, 2003) are recognized as important with regard to physical activity and exercise.

The unpleasant sensations that older adults can feel when performing a task have a major effect on their motivation. Most frequently identified among older adults are fear, pain, shortness of breath, and fatigue (Resnick & Spellbring, 2000; Yardley & Smith, 2002). Beliefs—in particular, individuals beliefs about what they are capable of doing and about the benefits of performing a given task—influence individuals' willingness to initiate and adhere to a specific activity (e.g., walking to the dining room). Social supports—family, peers, or clinical staff—also have influence motivation. Older adults, in particular, are eager to listen to and trust the recommendations and encouragement of clinicians such as physicians and nurses. Family, peers, and staff can impact motivation by providing verbal encouragement, helping to identify goals, and caring.

The importance of caring with regard to motivation should not be underestimated. Individuals who feel cared about, not just cared for, are generally more motivated to do what the caregiver requests them to do. Repeatedly, older adults report that they were motivated to perform activities because they felt cared for by a certain individual. Task performance is often the only thing older adults have to give back to the individual who demonstrated caring. Thus, older adults respond to the gift of caring with the gift of performing the requested task (Resnick & Spellbring, 2000).

Exposure to role models, can be very motivating for older adults, especially seeing similar individuals perform an activity. Seeing another older adult walk to the dining room when he or she used to be wheeled there, for example, motivates other individuals to do the same. This is particularly true if the role model is known to be older or perceived to have more debilitating illness (e.g., visible arthritis or neurological impairments) than the individual who is observing.

Ongoing verbal encouragement and reinforcement can be an important source of motivation, especially if provided by a trusted and respected individual. Caregivers can verbally encourage older adults when they work together with them to identify goals. Goal identification lets older adults know that the caregiver believes in their ability to perform the task associated with the goal. Encouragement and reinforcement also help to convey a sense of caring and make the individual feel cared about. Daily verbal encouragement to walk to the dining room reminds the older adult that the caregiver cares enough about him or her to continue providing that encouragement. Eventually the older adult may want to reciprocate and respond to the caregiver's efforts by walking. The motivational work does not end there, however. Once the behavior is performed, it is equally important to provide positive reinforcement for that behavior. Caregivers should not be afraid to get excited with older adults and openly show their excitement for even the smallest task accomplished. The older adult's participation—in bathing and/or in walking into the bathroom—should be followed by praise, a hug, a smile, and further encouragement.

One of the most important factors that influence motivation is prior experience of successful performance of the activity. Therefore, one of the best interventions to motivate and increase motivation is to help the older adult successfully perform a given activity. With any activity, initiation and performing it for the first time are the most difficult (e.g., the first day of starting an exercise program, quitting smoking, or going on a diet). Once some success is experienced, however, individuals have increased confidence in their ability to perform the activity. As their confidence increases, they will be more likely to perform the activity.

The factors identified in the Wheel of Motivation are consistent with social cognitive theory and the theory of self-efficacy as described in chapter 1. Social cognitive theory states that individuals, their environment, and their experiences interact to influence motivation. In this concept, motivation is viewed as dynamic. Personality may play an important part in the individual's behavior; however, health care providers can use interventions to strengthen or decrease motivation.

THE MOTIVATIONAL IMPACT OF ENVIRONMENT

Older adults are greatly influenced by the environment in which they live. Traditionally, a move into a long-term care facility has been associated with a decline in function and a need for 24-hour nursing care or supervision. Moreover, these facilities are commonly associated with end of life, death, and further decline. These beliefs may be confirmed by older adults, since 75% of individuals in long-term care settings need assistance with three or more activities of daily living (Department of Health and Human Services, 1999). The physical environment in long-term care facilities, of course, may vary greatly, but some common features of long-term care facilities can have a positive impact on function, particularly when compared to the home environment. For example, safety is a primary interest in long-term care, and consequently these facilities tend to have flat hallways with rails, which potentially can serve as an impetus to ambulate, at least for short functional distances.

Unfortunately, however, in long-term care settings nurses and nursing assistants are available 24-hours a day to provide care. The nursing care can, in some cases, create dependency (Beck et al., 1997; Davies, Ellis, & Laker, 2000; Resnick, 1998; 1999a and b; Waters, 1994) and be a significant factor in causing functional impairment in older adults in long-term care settings. Older adults who have someone available to perform a task for them can become less motivated to engage in care activities that might help them maintain and/or improve function.

Assisted Living

Assisted living facilities, based on a Scandinavian model of care, were developed to offer older adults both independence and a sense of community (National Center for Assisted Living, 2001). These settings emphasize offering choice in personal care and health-related services. Overall, individuals in these settings are less functionally impaired than those in long-term care settings (National Center for Assisted Living, 2001). Although the availability of staff and the cost of performing specific care activities for residents varies among assisted living settings, the staffing ratios are lower than in long-term care facilities, and caregivers are therefore generally less available. In these facilities older adults have less help available, and they also may be more motivated to engage in functional activities so they may remain in the facility indefinitely. Assisted living, like long-term care, also may provide a safe physical environment conducive to performing functional activities, such as walking in uncluttered hallways or bathing in large bathrooms with handrails.

Home Setting

The home setting, particularly for older adults who live alone or who do not have a caregiver readily available, may provide an environment that helps to motivate the individual to perform necessary functional activities. Activities of daily living, such as bathing and dressing, and instrumental activities of daily living, such as taking medications, cooking, or washing clothes, must be performed at some level in order to survive. Services can be paid for, although this help has a significant cost over time. In addition, some older adults are not willing to have strangers enter their home to perform activities. In order to survive in the home setting, older adults are motivated to perform. Conversely, however, the environment in some home settings may decrease motivation to perform functional activities and exercise. Stairs, for example, may not be well lit, may be in poor condition, and/or may not have handrails. The home setting also may not have flat, open, uncluttered areas in which to walk. This environment can decrease the older adult's confidence to perform activities such as distance ambulation or stair climbing.

SPECIAL MOTIVATION ISSUES IN COGNITIVELY IMPAIRED OLDER ADULTS

Little is known about motivation in individuals with cognitive impairment. Unfortunately, these individuals may be labeled as unmotivated when, in fact, they are resisting care because of fear in unfamiliar situations or lack of confidence to perform the suggested behavior. These individuals may cope with a given care-related situation by using strategies such as attaining control, sharing control, or resigning control to the caregiver, or they may cope by regaining their own inner control (Kovach & Meyer-Arnold, 1996). Caregivers may interpret a decline in function and loss of communication associated with cognitive impairment to be equivalent to helplessness and an inability to perform simple functional tasks (Bootsma-van der Wiel et al., 2001; Vogelpohl, Beck, Heacock & Mercer, 1996). The tendency may be to simply provide total care to these individuals, resulting in further loss of independence and greater functional decline.

There is a known discrepancy in older adults with cognitive impairment between ability to perform a given task and the actual performance of that task (Bootsma-van der Wiel et al., 2001; Vogelpohl et al., 1996). These individuals are often capable of performing a specific activity of daily living but do not perform it. Some of this problem is likely iatrogenic, that is, caused by caregivers providing total care. Some, however, is due to motivation and a progressive decline in the individuals' beliefs about their abilities (Resnick, 1999a and b).

Vogelpohl and colleagues (1996) described strategies to promote independence in dressing among older adults with cognitive impairment. These strategies match the level of assistance provided with the person's cognitive and physical abilities and disabilities. Attempts are made to look beyond the older adult's usual level of functional performance to identify and mobilize underlying cognitive and physical reserves and maximize the individual's functional capacity. In addition to assessing the individual carefully to best identify underlying ability and capacity, as described in chapter 3, general care strategies can be used to fa-

TABLE 5.6   Strategies to Promote Independent Function in Cognitively Impaired Older Adults

1. Establish a routine that provides structure and decreases stress.
2. Be flexible and sensitive to fluctuations in cognition.
3. Modify the environment to augment function and decrease distractions.
4. Establish a routine consistent with prior life experiences (e.g., coffee before bathing).
5. Maintain a calm, loving, relaxed, unhurried manner during care interactions.
6. Provide verbal prompting with simple one-step commands and repetition.
7. Augment verbal cueing with gestures and modeling.
8. Provide positive reinforcement for desired behavior.

cilitate functional performance. These strategies are described in Table 5.6.

USING MOTIVATIONAL INTERVENTIONS TO AUGMENT FUNCTION

Using social cognitive theory and the theory of self-efficacy as a framework, a standardized intervention can be implemented to motivate older adults in any setting to engage in restorative care activities. Older adults are a heterogeneous group, and some interventions may be more effective with certain individuals than others. However, the interventions generally will increase the likelihood of helping these individuals achieve and maintain their highest level of function.

The interventions' focus is on building the self-efficacy and outcome expectations of older adults. Strengthening older adults' beliefs in their ability to perform a functional task and their beliefs about the benefit of performance will increase their willingness to engage in the activity over time. The four informational sources that influence self-efficacy and outcome expectations are used. These include verbal encouragement, decreasing unpleasant sensations (i.e., affective or physiological state), role modeling or self-modeling, and performance accomplishment.

Verbal Encouragement Through Education and Goal Setting

The outcomes of behavior are particularly important to older adults (Resnick, Palmer, Jenkins & Spellbring,

What Is Restorative Care?

Restorative nursing care focuses on the restoration and/or maintenance of physical function and helps older adults to perform their own personal activities such as bathing, dressing, and walking and other daily exercise and encourages them to do as much as possible for themselves.

Restorative care focuses on preventing disability and helping you improve and maintain your physical and psychological health so that you can continue to function as independently as possible.

What Can Restorative Care Do?
- Improve strength and maximum aerobic capacity
- Prevent disease
- Decrease your risk of falling

Restorative Care Activities

Participating in personal care activities can
- strengthen your muscles and bones
- improve your flexibility
- improve your overall feeling of well-being

Increase your activity by
- decreasing time spent in a wheelchair
- walking to the bathroom or dining room
- doing as much of your own personal care as possible

Incorporate exercise into your daily activity:
- Move yourself around in bed.
- Get up and down from the bed or chair frequently (every half hour).
- Walk instead of using the wheelchair.
- Participate in daily activities.

Overcome the Challenges to Performing Restorative Care Activities

Do you feel that you don't have enough time?
- Relax! There is no rush to get these activities done.

Do you feel too tired to exercise or perform personal care?
- The activity will give you energy. Try it and see!

Do you have too much pain to exercise or perform personal care activities?.
- Pain medication and other treatments can help control pain to get you started. And exercise can help prevent future pain.

Are you worried about getting hurt?
- The exercises and activities given to you are ones that you can do safely. Exercise will strengthen you.

FIGURE 5.2   Motivational poster.

2000). Therefore, it is essential to help them understand, through appropriate education, the many benefits of performing functional activities. The education component recommended includes using a easy-to-understand booklet, "Maintaining Function and Health," or the "Maintaining Function and Health" poster (Figure 5.2). The booklet reviews the benefits of participating in functional activities and exercise for older adults in long-term care settings, lists the challenges of participating in functional activities, and describes ways to overcome the challenges. The caregiver—nursing assistant, family member, nurse, or other provider—can review the poster or booklet during care activities. Regular repetition of the information is essential.

Individuals who are encouraged verbally and assured that they are capable of performing an activity are more likely to perform it. Table 5.7 provides examples of verbal encouragement dos and don'ts. Specifically, verbal encouragement should be realistic, should focus on positive information even if this is just small achievements, and should be given in such a way as to demonstrate caring. Individuals who are rewarded with positive verbal reinforcement following

an activity are more likely to continue to perform the given activity.

Identifying and setting goals with an individual is another useful way to provide verbal encouragement. Setting goals with individuals lets them know that the caregiver believes in their ability to perform the activity. The verbal encouragement intervention should include initial goal identification with the older adult and continued verbal encouragement to reinforce progress toward set goals. The champion of the

TABLE 5.7   Verbal Encouragement Dos and Don'ts

1. Use encouragement that is realistic and honest.
2. Demonstrate caring through your encouragement by looking the individual in the eye and letting him or her know how sincerely happy, proud, thrilled you are about his or her behavior.
3. Focus on the positive, and reinforce any and all positive exercise behavior. For example, if a participant didn't achieve her goal but exercised for part of the time, tell her how great it was that she exercised that much time, and let her know that next week you believe she will make the full 20 minutes.
4. Demonstrate your competence and expertise in exercise benefits and in evaluating outcomes. This will increase the credibility of your verbal encouragement.

restorative care program and a nursing assistant or caregiver who has worked with the older adult should talk with the older adult and identify daily short-term goals. Short-term goals generally are to perform a specific functional activity or participate in a simple exercise program. Long-term goals also should be identified and will vary based on what is relevant to the individual (e.g., walking to the dining room for all three meals or being able to go on a trip, go out with family, or lift a grandchild). Goals can be written on a special Goal Identification Form and placed in the older adult's room on the bullentin board, closet, or wall.

During daily encounters, the nursing assistants or caregiver can talk with the older adult about progress toward goals. Any progress toward goal attainment should be acknowledged. As previously discussed, letting older adults know how genuinely happy you are about their progress is a great way to encourage ongoing involvement in the activity. Following restorative care activities, the nursing assistant and/or the champion of the restorative care program can routinely give a hug, cheer, clap, and/or sit down and spend some time visiting with the older adult as a way to reward the behavior and goal achievement.

Goals should be evaluated at regular intervals and can be revised as appropriate. Monthly intervals may be sufficient, although this may vary based on the individual. In addition, a review of progress toward identified goals reminds older adults of what they have successfully performed and therefore strengthens self-efficacy and outcome expectations.

Decreasing Unpleasant Sensations

Decreasing unpleasant sensations associated with activities can help motivate older adults. Older adults do not want to engage in an activity that is unpleasant (Resnick, 1998; 1999a and b; Resnick & Spellbring, 2000). Consequently, unpleasant sensations should be eradicated when older individuals perform functional activities or exercise. The best ways to determine if the older adult is experiencing unpleasant sensations during an activity are to observe performance and/or ask the individual. Older adults' most common complaints associated with functional tasks and exercise include pain, fear, fatigue, boredom, or shortness of breath. Table 5.8 provides examples of ways to evaluate older individuals for evidence of these problems. Additional unpleasant sensations to consider include feelings of fullness with eating, cramping associated with walking, or embarrassment of being seen with disabilities and having to use assistive devices. Nursing assistants, nurses, and other caregivers should discuss any unpleasant sensations identified by older adults and to encourage them to give a reason or rationale for why they do not want to do an activity. This information should then be addressed by establishing a plan of care to decrease those sensations.

Interventions to decrease unpleasant sensations such as pain, fear, fatigue, shortness of breath, and boredom can be initiated by nursing assistants or other caregivers and should be developed in conjunction with other members of the health care team as appropriate (see Appendix).

TABLE 5.8   Identifying Unpleasant Sensations

Unpleasant Sensation	Measurement Techniques or Tools
Pain	Checklist for the Presence of Pain (Table 5.8a) Numeric Pain Scale (Table 5.8b) Pain Description (Table 5.8b)
Fear	Rating of fear on a 0 to 4 scale 0 1 2 3 4 no fear a lot of fear
Shortness of breath	Direct observation Pulse oximetry to determine oxygen levels as cause of shortness of breath Deconditioning as cause of shortness of breath (Table 5.8c)

TABLE 5.8a   Checklist for the Presence of Pain

_____ Frowning, grimacing, fearful facial expression, grinding of teeth
_____ Bracing, guarding or rubbing body part
_____ Fidgeting, increasing or recurring agitation
_____ Striking out, increasing or recurring agitation
_____ Eating or sleeping poorly
_____ Sighing, groaning, crying, breathing heavily—especially with movement
_____ Decreased activity from usual
_____ Resistance of certain movements such as lifting an arm
_____ Change in gait, with difficulty bearing weight
_____Change in function
_____Verbal expression or complaint of pain upon questioning

TABLE 5.8b   Pain Assessment

Numeric Scale for Pain
Pain Intensity:
How bad is your pain right now?

0	1	2	3	4	5	6	7	8	9	10
no pain										severe pain

Pain Description
Pattern: Constant Intermittent
Duration:_____
Location:_____
Character:
   Burning
   Shooting
   Stinging
   Tingling
   Sharp
   Radiating or moving
Things that make pain worse: _____
_____
_____

Things that make pain better: _____
_____
_____

Interventions to Decrease Pain

Nursing assistants and other caregivers should inform nursing staff in the facility, or the older adult's primary care provider if in the home setting, about any complaints or observations that indicate the individual is experiencing pain. The nurse or primary care provider can then review current treatments and determine if these treatments are being used, if medications are managing the pain at optimal usage, and if they are being used appropriately. For example, it may be best to coordinate timing of pain medication with restorative care activities (i.e., half an hour before treatment). Other treatment options include using complementary

TABLE 5.8c   Checklist for Evidence of Deconditioning

____ A reduction in cardiorespiratory endurance, and dyspnea and fatigue occurring earlier during aerobic exercise
____ Heart rate elevated at rest and increases markedly during submaximal levels of exercise
____ Atrophy of the skeletal muscles
____ Decline in muscle strength and endurance due to loss of muscle mass
____ Worsening of motor control and balance
____ Slower reaction times

techniques to decrease pain, such as heat and ice over a sore joint or muscle, relaxation techniques such as deep breathing and visual imagery to decrease pain, and appropriate positioning. Staff also should remind older adults that exercise and activity are often the best way to decrease pain, particularly for some types of musculoskeletal discomfort. These pain-relieving techniques should be taught to nursing assistants or care providers during the recommended 6-week education sessions (chapter 2).

Interventions to Decrease Fear of Falling or Getting Hurt

Nursing assistants, nurses, and other caregivers should expect that older adults, particularly those who have experienced a fall, may have some fear of falling or getting hurt. This is true even in those with memory impairment. These individuals may not remember the fall or the experiences around the fall, but they remember the feeling associated with the fall, that is, the fea. Explore these feelings of fear by encouraging the older adults to talk about the fear. Help them to feel comfortable expressing this fear, and explore the depth and degree to which it stops them from doing activities.

Interventions to decrease fear include reinforcing to the individuals *repeatedly* that they will not be asked to do any activities that are not safe for them. More importantly, teach older adults that the best way to prevent a fall and getting hurt is to be active and exercise to strengthen muscles and bones. The 6-week educational sessions described in chapter 2 teach nursing assistants and care providers the skills and confidence to perform restorative care activities. This competence must be demonstrated to older adults so that they feel secure in the caregiver's ability to help with functional activities.

Once it becomes evident that an older adult has fear associated with an activity, caregivers should focus on building confidence about that activity, and thereby decreasing the fear. Confidence increases through meeting small goals that build up to the full activity. For example, the older individual may be afraid of walking to the bathroom from bed. The goals could start with sitting up independently and coming to a stand at the edge of the bed for a few minutes. The length of time standing could then increase. The next goal could be to take a couple of steps in place and then sit back down. This could progress to taking several steps forward. Ultimately, the goal would be to walk to the bathroom. At this point, with much encouragement and support, the individual will have confidence and feel safe and comfortable walking the distance to the bathroom.

Interventions to Manage Fatigue

Older adults also commonly experience fatigue associated with physical activity, and this should be anticipated. Fatigue may occur for numerous reasons, including poor sleep, disease, medication side effects, or excessive activity (i.e., in wanderers). Caregivers in any setting should schedule rest periods to augment restorative care time. Rest periods can even be a way to motivate the individual to do restorative care activities. For example, a promised nap can be very effective before walking to the dining room for dinner or sitting with the family at the dinner table. This kind of care requires a good deal of flexibility, especially in institutional settings. Restorative care activities, however, cannot be forced into specific time blocks but must occur at a mutually acceptable time. Negotiating and planning rest periods for restorative care is a great way to build in that flexibility. Reinforce to the older adult that activity and exercise are important interventions that can directly decrease fatigue. This is particularly true if the fatigue is due to boredom or disease states (physical and or emotional).

Interventions to Decrease Sensations of Shortness of Breath

When developing and implementing a restorative care program for an older adult, nursing staff, nursing assistants, and other care providers should determine if shortness of breath is generally present in the individual. In addition, all caregivers should be asked if the shortness of breath is exacerbated following the initiation of restorative care activities. Shortness of breath may be due to disease states such as chronic obstructive pulmonary disease (COPD), heart failure, or lung cancer, or it may be due simply to deconditioning. In the institutional or home setting, attempt to establish if the older adult needs supplemental oxygen by checking simple pulse oximetry. Testing should be done while the older individual is performing restorative care activities such as bathing, dressing, eating, or am-

bulating. A pulse oximetry that drops below 90 during these activities indicates a need for supplemental oxygen at least during the activity. This information should be discussed with the older individual's primary care provider.

Once the cause of the shortness of breath is identified, the appropriate treatment plan can be initiated. Certainly, older adults who need oxygen should be supplied with and encouraged to use oxygen during activity. Some older adults are embarrassed to be seen with oxygen and refuse to use it when out in public. Caregivers should anticipate this resistance and repeatedly work with older individuals to increase their understanding of the importance of oxygen when performing activities. For older individuals who become short of breath due to deconditioning, caregivers should provide sufficient time to rest between steps in completion of the activity. In addition, individuals with COPD should be taught pursed lip breathing to improve oxygen exchange (Table 5.9).

Interventions to Make Activity/Exercise Less Boring and More Fun

Many older adults did not incorporate exercise into daily activities when they were younger and did not

TABLE 5.9 Pursed Lip Breathing Exercises

Technique
1. Relax your neck and shoulder muscles.
2. Breathe in (inhale) slowly through your nose for two counts, keeping your mouth closed. Don't take a deep breath. A normal breath will do. It may help to count to yourself: inhale, one, two.
3. Pucker or "purse" your lips as if you were going to whistle or gently flicker the flame of a candle.
4. Breathe out (exhale) slowly and gently through your pursed lips while counting to four. It may help to count to yourself: exhale, one, two, three, four.

Purpose
- Improves ventilation
- Releases trapped air in the lungs
- Keeps the airways open longer and decreases the work of breathing
- Prolongs exhalation to slow the breathing rate
- Improves breathing patterns by moving old air out of the lungs and allowing for new air to enter the lungs
- Relieves shortness of breath
- Causes general relaxation

use leisure time to exercise. For many of these individuals, activity and exercise are seen as boring. Consider motivational interventions to make the activity less boring and more fun. An art gallery to view pictures on the way to the dining room, walking in a group with others to talk with, and laughing and joking during an activity are all ways to make activities fun. These activities can be effective even for those with memory impairment because, although they may not remember the activity, they will remember the pleasant sensations of fun that went along with it.

Role-Modeling or Self-Modeling

Exposing older adults to role models, or like individuals performing a given activity, may or may not serve as a motivational intervention. Some older adults report that seeing people who are similar to them in age, health, and physical ability successfully perform an activity helps them to believe that they also can do the activity. Other older adults report that what others do has no impact on what they feel they are capable of doing or are willing to do. Explore with older adults how it makes them feel to see their roommates walk to the dining room or out in the hallway, or how it makes them feel if someone else falls or gets hurt doing an activity. Depending on the response of the individual, exposure to role models can be used.

In group settings such as small exercise classes, role models are often effective. This is particularly true for individuals with some cognitive impairment because the role model can be pointed to as motivation to do the same activity. Seeing another older adult using an exercise band or handheld weight successfully during exercise class, for example, can motivate other members of the class to do the same.

Self-modeling may be an even more consistent way to motivate older individuals who tend to focus on their own personal progress, condition, and physical needs. Self-modeling helps remind individuals of their capabilities to perform specific activities, and thereby motivates them to continue to perform. In addition, cueing with self-modeling is an excellent source of motivation because the individual gets the verbal encouragement of the cueing and has help to know what he or she should be doing. The cues can serve as a reminder for the individual that he or she is capable of doing the activity required and has done so successfully in the past.

Cueing with self-modeling can be implemented by giving a monthly calendar to each older adult and placing this in a commonly viewed area of the room (e.g., door or bulletin board). The calendar can be marked off to remind the participant what type of activity to do each day (e.g., bathing upper extremity, walking to the dining room). The nursing assistant or other caregiver can be instructed to record the type of restorative care activity completed and the amount of time it took to complete. Seeing this information recorded reminds the older adult that he or she is capable of completing daily restorative care activities and serves as a cue to actually perform them. Cueing will also facilitate communication between nursing assistants and other caregivers so that everyone who provides care to the individual can facilitate the older individual's performance of restorative care activities.

Another fun and effective way to provide self-modeling and cueing is to take pictures of the older adult participating in restorative care activities, such as walking to the dining room, eating independently with assistive devices, or participating in an exercise class. These pictures can be placed on a bulletin board in the home or facility setting and updated as appropriate. The pictures can be used to remind the older individual of how he or she has progressed.

USING THE THREE Rs: RECOGNITION, REINFORCEMENT, AND REWARD

Recognizing individuals for what they are able and willing to do functionally is essential. For example, getting excited that an individual walked five steps to the bathroom or independently washed his or her upper extremity is very effective in maintaining performance of that activity. Positive feedback, praise, and hugs for all attempts to participate in functional activities are necessary to encourage continuation of these behaviors. This reinforcement should be realistic and honest. Care providers should demonstrate that they care by looking the older individual in the eye and letting him or her know how sincerely happy, proud, and thrilled they are about a given behavior or activity. Reinforcing beliefs about the individual's ability to perform the specific behavior of interest and about the benefits of performing that behavior are also necessary to help maintain the behavior.

Identifying appropriate rewards for older adults may be challenging. Be creative in the establishment of rewards. Going out with families or being ready for a visit with friends are wonderful rewards for performance of functional tasks. In addition, health care providers should use themselves as a reward: Give a hug and a kiss for behavior well done, or spend some extra time just visiting with the older individual.

CONCLUSION

Participation in restorative care activities, especially functional activities and physical activity and exercise, is often driven by the older adult's motivation. Some individuals are driven by an inner desire to get stronger, maintain health and function, and engage in regular physical activity. Some older adults with significant chronic medical problems, such as degenerative joint disease that limits the individual's ability to range his or her shoulders, will insist on bathing or dressing themselves on a daily basis. Another individual with the same medical problems may refuse to even attempt participate in bathing and dressing. These differences are due to personality. This chapter demonstrates that there are many interventions that health care providers can and should use to motivate older adults to engage in functional activities. The inner drive or motivation to perform functional skills is a very useful aspect of motivation. It is not, however, present in all individuals. Certainly, some older individuals are not motivated to engage in restorative care activities. The tendency among health care providers is to give up and perform the necessary care. The real challenge, however, is to use the techniques recommended in this chapter to motivate individuals to engage in restorative care activities at their highest possible level of involvement.

REFERENCES

Aller, L., & Coeling, H. (1995). Quality of life: Its meaning to the long-term care resident. *Journal of Gerontological Nursing, 21*(2), 20–25.

Beck, C., Heacock, P., Mercer, S., Walls, R., Rapp, C., & Vogelpohl, T. (1997). Improving dressing behavior in cognitively impaired nursing home residents. *Nursing Research, 46*(3), 126–132.

Berger, A.K., Fratiglioni, L., & Forsell, Y. (1999). The occurrence of depressive symptoms in the preclinical phase of AD: A population-based study. *Neurology, 53,* 1998–2002.

Bootsma-van der Wiel, A., Gussekloo, J., De Craen, A., Van Exel, E., Knook, D., Lagaay, A., & Westendorp, R. (2001). Disability in the oldest old: "Can do" or "do do"? *Journal of the American Geriatrics Society, 49,* 909–914.

Davies, S., Ellis, L., & Laker, S. (2000). Promoting autonomy and independence for older people within nursing practice: An observational study. *Journal of Clinical Nursing, 9,* 127–136.

Department of Health and Human Services. (1999). National nursing home survey. *Vital and Health Statistics.* Series 13, 152.

Jette, A., Rooks, D., Lachman, M., Lin, T., Levenson, C. Heislein, D., Giorgetti, M., & Harris, B. (1998). Home-based resistance training: Predictors of participation and adherence. *The Gerontologist, 38,* 412–421.

Kemp, B. (1988). Motivation, rehabilitation and aging: A conceptual model. *Topics in Geriatric Rehabilitation, 3*(3), 41–52.

Kovach, C.R., & Meyer-Arnold, E.A. (1996). Coping with conflicting agendas: The bathing experience of cognitively impaired older adults. *Scholarly Inquiry of Nursing Practice, 10*(1), 23–36; discussion 37–42.

MacRae, P., Asplund, L., Schnelle, J., Cheslande, J., Abrahmse, A., & Morris, C. (1996). A walking program for nursing home residents: Effects in walking endurance, physical activity, mobility and quality of life. *Journal of the American Geriatrics Society, 47,* 175–80.

Mulrow, C., Chiodu, L., Gerety, M., Lee, S., Basu, S., Nelson, D. (1996). Function and medical comorbidity in South Texas nursing home residents: variation by ethnic group. *Journal of the American Geiatrics Society, 44,* 279–284.

National Center for Assisted Living. (2001). Facts and trends. *The assisted living sourcebook* (5th ed.). Washington. DC.

Rejeski, W., & Brawley, L. (1997). Shaping active lifestyles in older adults: A group facilitated behavior change intervention. *Annals of Behavioral Medicine, 19*(Suppl), S106.

Resnick, B. (1996). Motivation in geriatric rehabilitation. *Image: The Journal of Nursing Scholarship, 28,* 41–47.

Resnick, B. (1998). Efficacy beliefs in geriatric rehabilitation. *Journal of Gerontological Nursing, 24,* 34–45.

Resnick, B. (1999a). Motivation in the older adult: can a leopard change its spots? *Journal of Advanced Nursing, 29,* 792–799.

Resnick, B. (1999b). Reliability and validity testing of the self-efficacy for functional activities scale. *Journal of Nursing Measurement, 7*(1), 5–20.

Resnick, B. (2000). Functional performance and exercise of older adults in long term care. *Journal of Gerontological Nursing, 26*(3), 7–16.

Resnick, B., Palmer, M.H., Jenkins, L., & Spellbring, A.M. (2000). Path analysis of efficacy expectations and exercise behavior in older adults. *Journal of Advanced Nursing, 31*(6), 1309–1315.

Resnick, B., & Spellbring, A.M. (2000). Understanding what motivates older adults to exercise. *Journal of Gerontological Nursing, 26*(3), 34–42.

Saelens, B.E., Sallis, J.F, & Frank, L.D. (2003). Environmental correlates of walking and cycling: Findings from the transportation, urban design, and planning literature. *Annals of Behavioral Medicine, 25*(2), 80–91.

The Senior Care Source. (2003). Facts, figures & forecasts. Novartis, East Hanover, .

Vogelpohl, T., Beck, C., Heacock, P., & Mercer, S. (1996). I can do it dressing: Promoting independence through individualized strategies. *Journal of Gerontological Nursing, 22*(3), 39–42.

Waters, K. (1994). Getting dressed in the early morning: Styles of staff/patient interaction on rehabilitation hospital wards for elderly people. *Journal of Advanced Nursing, 19,* 239–247.

Yardley, L., & Smith, H. (2002). A prospective study of the relationship between feared consequences of falling and avoidance of activity in community-living older people. *Gerontologist, 42*(1), 17–23.

CHAPTER 6

Documentation and Reimbursement for Restorative Care

Annette Fleishell

OVERVIEW

In any care setting, documentation of services and care provided is an important aspect of providing exemplary care, meeting state and federal care requirements, and capturing appropriate reimbursement for services provided. With regard to restorative care activities, documentation of services has been particularly sparse because the focus of health care is generally on negative events and/or documentation of changes in an older adult's physical condition and/or emotional state. The purpose of this chapter is to provide an understanding of the regulations related to restorative care activities and the impact of those regulations on documentation of services and reimbursement of restorative care. Examples of documentation tools are provided that can facilitate the documentation process and help facilities adhere to regulations and optimize reimbursement for restorative care services.

REGULATIONS FOR LONG-TERM CARE FACILITIES

As previously indicated, restorative care nursing was initially developed for long-term care settings. With passage of the Omnibus Budget Reconciliation Act (OBRA) of 1987, skilled nursing facilities became responsible for maintaining residents at their highest practicable level. Medicare and Medicaid Requirements for Long Term Care Facilities at F 309 (Centers for Medicare and Medicaid Services State Operations Manual, Appendix B, 1987) says, "Each resident must receive and the facility must provide the necessary care and services to attain or maintain the highest practicable physical, mental, and psychosocial well-being, in accordance with the comprehensive assessment and plan of care." "Highest practicable" is defined as the highest level of functioning and well-being possible, limited only by the individual's presenting functional status and potential for improvement or reduced rate of functional decline. This is determined through a comprehensive resident assessment by competently and thoroughly addressing the physical, mental, and psychosocial needs of the individual. The facility must ensure that the resident obtains optimal improvement or does not deteriorate, within the limits of a resident's right to refuse treatment and within the limits of recognized pathology and the normal aging process. In any instance when there has been a lack of improvement or a decline, the regulatory survey team must determine if the occurrence was unavoidable or avoidable. This determination can only be made if there is (1) an accurate and complete assessment of the older individual, (2) a care plan that is implemented consistently and is based on information from the assessment, and (3) an evaluation of the results of the interventions and documentation of appropriate revisions of the interventions (Health Care Financing Administration, 1999)

The federal requirements (Centers for Medicare and Medicaid Services State Operations Manual, Appendix B, 1987) further mandate, based on F 310, that "a resident's abilities in activities of daily living (Table 6.1) do not diminish unless circumstances of the indi-

TABLE 6.1 Activities of Daily Living as Defined by Federal Regulations

Bathe, dress, and groom
Transfer and ambulate
Toilet
Eat
Use speech, language, or other functional communication systems

TABLE 6.2 Components of Restorative Care Nursing Programs

- Ambulation and range of motion
- Maintaining good body alignment and proper positioning of bedbound residents
- Encouraging and assisting patients to change positions at least every 2 hours to stimulate circulation and prevent decubiti and deformities
- Encouraging and assisting patients to keep active and out of bed for reasonable periods of time, within the limitations permitted by physician's orders, and encouraging patients to achieve independence in activities
- Assisting patients to adjust to their disabilities, to use their prosthetic and assistive devices, and to redirect their interests, if necessary

vidual's clinical condition demonstrate that diminution was unavoidable."

The Centers for Medicare & Medicaid Services (CMS, formerly Health Care Financing Administration) have never mandated that facilities have nursing rehabilitation/restorative care programs. The intent, however, of the previously quoted regulation clearly identifies that the facility is responsible for providing programs that will not only maintain but also improve resident function, as indicated by the resident's comprehensive assessment and plan of care.

Since individual state regulations may supersede the federal statutes (providing they are more stringent), a formalized restorative care program may be required in any particular state. For instance, the Code of Maryland Regulations (COMAR) 10.07.02 for Comprehensive Care Facilities and Extended Care Facilities is specific in its requirements (COMAR, 1998). COMAR 10.07.02.12S mandates the development of a "Program of Restorative Nursing Care." Specifically, the recommendations state that there shall be an active program of restorative nursing care aimed at assisting each patient to achieve and maintain his highest level of individual function, including activities of daily living. Components of what should be included in this program are delineated in Table 6.2.

The *Scope and Standards of Gerontological Nursing Practice* (American Nurses Association, 2000) also describes nurses' responsibility to provide restorative care and services at Standard V, Planning and Continuity of Care: "The nurse develops the plan of care in conjunction with the older person and appropriate others. Mutual goals, priorities, nursing approaches, and measures in the care plan address the therapeutic, preventive, restorative, and rehabilitative needs of the older person. Implementation of the care plan should help the older person attain and maintain the highest level of health, well-being, and quality of life achievable."

Given the federal and state statutory requirements,

together with professionally identified standards of care, most facilities have found that the establishment of a structured restorative care program offers the best opportunity not only to attain, maintain, and slow decline of residents' function but also to satisfy documentation requirements for assessment, care planning, and evaluation (Fleishell, Mullins, & Watts, 2000)

Minimum Data Set Resident Assessment Documentation Requirements

OBRA has mandated a standardized comprehensive resident assessment, which was developed into the Minimum Data Set (MDS) 2.0. Requirements for timely completion of the comprehensive MDS assessment are also identified by OBRA (Table 6.3). MDS assessments are also required to be electronically submitted to the state agency when completed, according to CMS coding and editing requirements. These as-

TABLE 6.3 MDS Requirements for Documentation and Assessment

- Assessment must be done within 14 calendar days after admission.
- Assessment must be done within 14 days after the facility determines that there has been a significant change in the resident's physical or mental condition.
- Assessment must be done not less than every 12 months.
- A quarterly review assessment must be done not less frequently than every 3 months.

sessment requirements give a basic and minimum assessment tool for documentation of restorative nursing at certain sections of the MDS. The *Resident Assessment Instrument (RAI) User's Manual* (CMS, 1995) describes the intent of Section P3, Nursing Rehabilitation/Restorative Care, as follows: "To determine the extent to which the resident receives nursing rehabilitation or restorative services from other than specialized therapy staff (e.g., occupational therapist, physical therapist, etc.). Rehabilitative or restorative care refers to nursing interventions that promote the resident's ability to adapt and adjust to living as independently and safely as is possible. This concept actively focuses on achieving and maintaining optimal physical, mental, and psychosocial functioning. Skill practice in such activities as walking and mobility, dressing and grooming, eating and swallowing, transferring, amputation care, and communication can improve or maintain function in physical abilities and ADLs and prevent further impairment." Table 6.4 depicts the section of the MDS where restorative activities should be documented. The user's manual further defines each of these areas as shown in Table 6.5. Activities include such things as range of motion, transfers, ambulation, bathing, dressing, and training and skill practice interventions. These definitions of restorative care activities may differ from clinical and professional definitions, but are used specifically for MDS documentation and coding purposes. They should be incorporated into documentation requirements of the facility nursing restorative care program.

Adherence to the coding instructions is critical to accurate documentation on Section P3 of the MDS assessment: "Record the number of days each of the following rehabilitation or restorative techniques or practices was provided to the resident for more than or equal to 15 minutes per day in the last 7 days" (*MDS 2.0 User's Manual*, 2000). The 15 minutes does not have to occur all at once. Remember that persons with dementia learn skills best through repetition that occurs multiple times per day. It is important to review each activity throughout the 24-hour period. In order to comply with this coding requirement, an effective nursing restorative care program must use documentation tools that can capture this required information. Such tools may also be used to document restorative care activities that are not included in the MDS assessment categories. Tables 6.6 and 6.7 are sample documentation tools that fulfill documentation requirements for accurate coding of time spent on various restorative activities.

It is important to note that bowel and bladder retraining are, of themselves, not considered as nursing restorative care programs under Section P3 of the MDS, but rather should be coded in Section H3, Appliances and Programs (Table 6.8). Coding instructions for this section require a check in the appropriate item. Only items 3a, any scheduled toileting plan, and 3b, bladder retraining program, are considered to be restorative in nature. The user's manual defines these activities as described in Table 6.9.

PROVIDERS OF RESTORATIVE CARE SERVICES

Until the implementation of the Balanced Budget Act (BBA) in July 1997, nursing rehabilitation/restorative

---

TABLE 6.4   MDS Version 2.0 Special Treatment and Procedures

SECTION P. SPECIAL TREATMENTS AND PROCEDURES

3.	NURSING REHABILITATION/ RESTORATIVE CARE	Record the NUMBER OF DAYS each of the following rehabilitation or restorative techniques or practices was provided to the resident for more than or equal to 15 minutes per day in the last 7 days (Enter 0 if none or less than 15 minutes daily.)

a. Range of motion (passive)	f. Walking
b. Range of motion (active)	g. Dressing or grooming
c. Splint or brace assistance	h. Eating or swallowing
TRAINING AND SKILL PRACTICE IN:	i. Amputation/prosthesis care
d. Bed mobility	j. Communication
e. Transfer	k. Other

TABLE 6.5   MDS User's Manual Definition of Functional Activities

Functional Activity	Definition
Range of motion	The extend to which or the limits between which a part of the body can be moved around a fixed point, or joint. Range of motion exercise is a program of passive or active movements to maintain flexibility and useful motion in the joints of the body.
Active range of motion	Exercises performed by a resident with cueing or supervision by staff that are planned, scheduled, and documented in the clinical record
Splint or brace assistance	Assistance can be of two types: (1) where staff provide verbal and physical guidance and direction that teaches the resident how to apply, manipulate, and care for a brace or splint; or (2) where staff have a scheduled program of applying and removing a splint or brace, assess the resident's skin and circulation under the device and reposition the limb in correct alignment. These sessions are planned, scheduled, and documented in the clinical record.
Training and skill practice	Activities including repetition, physical or verbal cueing, and task sequencing provided by any staff or volunteer under the supervision of a licensed nurse.
Bed mobility	Activities used to improve or maintain the resident's self-performance in moving to and from a lying position, turning side to side, and positioning him- or herself in bed
Transfer	Activities used to improve or maintain the resident's self-performance of moving between surfaces or planes either with or without assistive devices
Walking	Activities used to improve or maintain the resident's self-performance in walking with or without assistive devices
Dressing and grooming	Activities used to improve or maintain the resident's self-performance in dressing and undressing, bathing and washing, and performing other personal hygiene tasks
Eating or swallowing	Activities used to improve or maintain the resident's self-performance in feeding him- or herself food and fluids, or activities used to improve or maintain the resident's ability to ingest nutrition and hydration by mouth
Amputation/ prosthesis care	Activities used to improve or maintain the resident's self-performance in putting on and removing a prosthesis, caring for the prosthesis, and providing appropriate hygiene at the site where the prosthesis attaches to the body
Communication	Activities used to improve or maintain the resident's self-performance in using newly acquired functional communication skills or assisting the resident in using residual communication skills and adaptive devices
Other	Any other activities used to improve or maintain the resident's self-performance in functioning, e.g., self-care for diabetic management, self-administration of medications, ostomy care

care programs were frequently developed and supervised by therapists and delivered by nursing assistants. The BBA effectively eliminated this practice because therapists' time under the prospective payment system (PPS) became more tightly regulated and scrutinized. CMS requires that nursing rehabilitation/restorative care be nursing driven, using the skills and expertise of a nurse to plan and implement care pathways for returning individuals to their highest practicable level of well-being. This care does not necessarily have to be provided by nurses and nurse assistants. Under the supervision of a licensed nurse, non-nursing staff members such as therapeutic recreation specialists, volunteers, and even family members can deliver care that qualifies in certain categories of restorative care. Nursing rehabilitation/restorative care places an important

emphasis on prevention of secondary sequelae of physical dependence, inactivity, and immobility. While cure or complete restoration of function may not be realistic, most residents in long-term care facilities can benefit from participation in a restorative care program, whether this benefit is psychological, physical, or both. Comprehensive restorative care programs not only benefit long-term care residents, but also meet federal licensing and compliance regulations. (Fleishell et al., 2000).

The *RAI User's Manual* (CMS, 1995) provides guidance for CMS requirements for nursing rehabilitation/restorative care programs. The criteria to be considered for inclusion in the MDS Section P3, Nursing Rehabilitation/Restorative Care, are delineated in Table 6.10.

TABLE 6.6   Restorative Care Flowsheet 1

Record the number of minutes each rehabilitation activity was provided to the resident.		1	2	3	4	5	6	7	8	9	10	11	12	13	14	15	16	17	18	19	20
Passive range of motion (You did it for the resident.)	11 pm–7 am																				
	7 am–3 pm																				
	3 pm–11 pm																				
Active range of motion (The resident participated in the activity.)	11 pm–7 am																				
	7 am–3 pm																				
	3 pm–11 pm																				
Application/removal of splint or brace Does resident assist? ☐ Yes ☐ No Does resident perform? ☐ Yes ☐ No	11 pm–7 am																				
	7 am–3 pm																				
	3 pm–11 pm																				
Amputation or prosthesis care Does resident assist? ☐ Yes ☐ No Does resident perform? ☐ Yes ☐ No	11 pm–7 am																				
	7 am–3 pm																				
	3 pm–11 pm																				
Eating/swallowing Special dining program? ☐ Yes ☐ No	11 pm–7 am																				
	7 am–3 pm																				
	3 pm–11 pm																				
Communication activity Practice area _____ Device used _____ Goal _____	11 pm–7 am																				
	7 am–3 pm																				
	3 pm–11 pm																				
Scheduled toileting plan:	11 pm–7 am																				
	7 am–3 pm																				
	3 pm–11 pm																				
Bladder retraining plan:	11 pm–7 am																				
	7 am–3 pm																				
	3 pm–11 pm																				

TABLE 6.7　Restorative Care Flowsheet 2

Record the number of minutes each rehabilitation activity was provided to the resident.		1	2	3	4	5	6	7	8	9	10	11	12	13	14	15	16	17	18	19	20
Bed Mobility	11 pm–7 am																				
Does resident assist?	7 am–3 pm																				
☐ Yes　　☐ No	3 pm–11 pm																				
Does resident perform?																					
☐ Yes　　☐ No																					
Goals: _____																					
Transfer	11 pm–7 am																				
Does resident assist?	7 am–3 pm																				
☐ Yes　　☐ No	3 pm–11 pm																				
Does resident perform?																					
☐ Yes　　☐ No																					
Goals: _____																					
Walking	11 pm–7 am																				
Does resident assist?	7 am–3 pm																				
☐ Yes　　☐ No	3 pm–11 pm																				
Does resident perform?																					
☐ Yes　　☐ No																					
Goals: _____																					
Dressing/Grooming	11 pm–7 am																				
Does resident assist?	7 am–3 pm																				
☐ Yes　　☐ No	3 pm–11 pm																				
Does resident perform?																					
☐ Yes　　☐ No																					
Goals: _____																					
Other: Refer to policy	11 pm–7 am																				
List activity	7 am–3 pm																				
_____	3 pm–11 pm																				
Identify goal																					
_____																					
Other: Refer to policy	11 pm–7 am																				
List activity	7 am–3 pm																				
_____	3 pm–11 pm																				
Identify goal																					
_____																					
Initials																						

TABLE 6.8   MDS Continence: Appliances and Programs

SECTION H. CONTINENCE IN LAST 14 DAYS						
3.	APPLIANCES AND PROGRAMS	Any scheduled toileting plan	a.	Did not use toilet room/commode/urinal	f.
		Bladder retraining program	b.	Pads/briefs used	g.
		External (condom) catheter	c.	Enemas/irrigation	h.
		Indwelling catheter	d.	Ostomy present	i.
		Intermittent catheter	e.	None of the above	j.
4.	CHANGE IN URINARY CONTINENCE	Resident's urinary continence has changed as compared to status of 90 days ago (or since last assessment if less than 90 days)			
		0. No change 1. Improved 2. Deteriorated			

*H3 a & b included in Nursing Rehab calculation

EXAMPLES OF NURSING REHABILITATION/RESTORATIVE CODING FOR MDS DOCUMENTATION

The following are examples of how to document and code for restorative care nursing services in the long-term care setting.

Mr. V has lost range of motion (ROM) in his right arm, wrist, and hand due to a cerebrovascular accident (CVA) experienced several years ago. He has moderate to severe loss of cognitive decision-making skills and memory. To avoid further ROM loss and contractures to his right arm, the occupational therapist fabricated a resting right-hand splint and developed instructions for its application and removal. The restorative nursing coordinator developed instructions for providing passive range of motion exercises to his

right arm, wrist, and hand three times per day. The nursing assistants and Mr. V's wife have been instructed on how and when to apply and remove the hand splint and how to do the passive range-of-motion exercises. These plans are documented on Mr. V's care plan. The total amount of time involved each day in applying and removing the hand splint and completing the ROM exercises is 30 minutes. The nursing assistants report that, when bathing or dressing Mr. V., there is less resistance in his affected extremity for both splint or brace assistance and ROM (passive). It is recommended that the nurse enter "7" as the number of days these nursing restorative techniques were provided (*MDS 2.0 User's Manual*, 2002).

Mrs. J had a CVA less than a year ago, resulting in left-sided hemiplegia. Mrs. J has a strong desire to participate in her own care. Although she cannot

TABLE 6.9   Definition of Activities Under Scheduled Toileting and Bladder Retraining Programs

Program	Definition
Scheduled toileting plan	A plan whereby staff members at scheduled times each day take the resident to the toilet room, give the resident a urinal, or remind the resident to go to the toilet. Includes habit training and/or prompted voiding.
Bladder retraining program	A retraining program where the resident is taught to consciously delay urinating or resist the urgency to void. Residents are encouraged to void on a schedule rather than according to their urge to void. This form of training is used to manage urinary incontinence due to bladder instability.

TABLE 6.10   CMS Criteria for Nursing Rehabilitation/Restorative Care

1. Measurable objectives and interventions must be documented in the care plan and in the clinical record.
2. Evidence of periodic evaluation by a licensed nurse must be present in the clinical record.
3. Nurse assistants/aides must be trained in the techniques that promote resident involvement in the activity.
4. These activities are carried out or supervised by members of the nursing staff. Sometimes under licensed nurse supervision, other staff and volunteers will be assigned to work with specific residents.
5. This category does not include exercise groups with more than four residents per supervising helper or caregiver.

dress herself independently, she is capable of participating in this activity of daily living (ADL). Mrs. J's overall care plan goal is to maximize her independence in ADLs. A plan, documented on the care plan, has been developed to teach Mrs. J how to put on and take off her blouse with no physical assistance from the staff. All of her blouses have been adapted for front closure with Velcro. The nursing assistants have been instructed in how to verbally guide Mrs. J as she puts on and takes off her blouse. It takes approximately 20 minutes per day for Mrs. J to complete this task (dressing and undressing). It is recommended that in this scenario the nurse enter "7" as the number of days training and skill practice for dressing and grooming was provided (*MDS 2.0 User's Manual,* 2002).

Mrs. K was admitted to the nursing facility 7 days ago following a repair to a fractured hip. Physical therapy was delayed due to complications and a weakened condition. Upon admission she had difficulty moving herself in bed and required total assistance for transfers. To prevent further deterioration and increase her independence, the nursing staff implemented a plan on the second day following admission to teach her how to move herself in bed and transfer from bed to chair using a trapeze, the bedrails, and a transfer board. The plan was documented in Mrs. K's clinical record and communicated to all staff at the change of shift. The charge nurse documented in the nurses' notes that in the five days that Mrs. K has been receiving training and skill practice in bed mobility and transferring, her endurance and strength are improving, and she requires only extensive assistance for transferring. Each day the amount of time to provide this nursing restorative intervention has been decreasing so that the past five days, the average time is 45 minutes. In this scenario it is recommended that the nurse enter "5" as the number of days training and skill practice for bed mobility and transfer was provided (*MDS 2.0 User's Manual,* 2002).

Mr. W's cognitive status has been deteriorating progressively over the past several months. Despite deliberate nursing restorative attempts to promote his independence in feeding himself, he will not eat unless fed. Mr. W did not receive nursing restorative care for eating in the last 7 days. In this final scenario it is recommended that the nurse enter "0" as the number of days training and skill practice for eating was provided (*MDS 2.0 User's Manual,* 2002).

SKILLED THERAPY AND NURSING RESTORATIVE CARE SERVICES

Although restorative care and rehabilitation overlap, there is a specific focus for each program. Rehabilitation focuses on retraining, education, and the teaching of skills, and results from an acute injury or episode. Rehabilitation is a task-oriented discipline with a specific aim to be achieved within a definite period of time.

Restorative nursing focuses on restoring or compensating for skills lost through disuse or changes in physiology. It is based on the nursing model with less continued direct input from formalized therapy. Restorative nursing seeks to maximize and prolong abilities with specific, measurable objectives and is a continuing process (Collard, 1998).

Nursing restorative care can be an important adjunct to skilled therapy interventions under both Part A and Part B of Medicare. At times, residents need to continue to practice tasks learned in skilled therapy in order to maintain or improve their ability to perform the task. Medicare does not consider skilled therapy necessary for task repetition; rather, it is one of the functions of nursing restorative care. For example, a resident may become independent in transfers before he can walk independently. In this case, the therapist may continue to work on those resident deficits requiring the therapist's expertise such as gait training, while the nursing restorative team works on repetition of transfers and begins to practice the gait training (Fleishell et al., 2000).

Skilled therapy may be required in some cases of functional decline. If a restorative care program fails to help the resident regain functional ability that was reasonably expected to improve, assessment and treatment by the rehabilitation staff may be indicated. Additionally, some cognitively impaired residents may require a brief period of occupational therapy (OT) to develop an appropriate functional maintenance program. When physical, occupational, or speech therapy is indicated, it is imperative to ensure that the nursing restorative and skilled therapy are providing complementary rather than duplicated services. If a fiscal intermediary determines that services were duplicated on a resident, the facility risks losing reimbursement for the skilled therapy (Fleishell et al., 2000).

Resident rehabilitation can easily be delivered by nursing restorative care and skilled therapy services working independently of one another. For example, a resident may have a decline in walking endurance after a urinary tract infection, and a nursing restorative ambulation program would appropriately address the problem without the intervention of physical therapy (PT). On the other hand, a resident with a massive stroke will begin walking in PT long before it is appropriate for the nursing staff to walk the resident. (Watts & Mullins, 2000). If the resident is at the end of specialized therapy sessions, the licensed nurse may consult with the therapist regarding the resident's deficit and develop a potential plan of treatment for a restorative program. The final therapy assessment done by the licensed therapist may be used as the initial assessment for planning the restorative care program for that resident.

A period of skilled therapy that addresses a particular deficit may be followed by a period of nursing restorative care to continue or maintain progress. For example, the OT may fabricate a splint to address a hand contracture. The OT could develop a range of motion and splinting program that the nursing restorative team will follow. This case demonstrates a time where the nursing restorative team follows the recommendation of the skilled therapist. Conversely, if the nursing restorative care team identifies a deficit and delivers care for a period of time without progress, an assessment by a member of the skilled rehabilitation team may be in order. For example, if a resident has demonstrated a decline in transfer abilities and a period of nursing restorative care fails to mitigate the problem, it would be appropriate for the physical therapist to assess the problem. The resident's documented lack of progress in spite of nursing restorative care is sound justification for skilled intervention (Watts & Mullins, 2000).

The nursing restorative team and skilled therapy may also work together to address deficits. A resident may have multiple deficits, some of which may be addressed by therapy only and some by nursing only. For example, a resident may be on grooming and bathing programs under the supervision of the nursing restorative team, while the OT might be working on dressing problems. Alternately, nursing and therapy may be working on different aspects of the same problem. For example, a resident with swallowing problems may be on a thickened liquid feeding program with the restorative nursing team, while the speech pathologist develops the resident's ability to tolerate thin liquids (Watts & Mullin, 2000).

What is essential in each of these scenarios is that the restorative team and the skilled therapist communicate well, work closely together, and agree on systems and procedures that will eliminate duplication of efforts and discrepancies in documentation, especially scoring on the MDS. Education, collaboration, and a planned communication system are essential for success. How nursing staff document each resident's progress (or lack of progress) will be critical to back up claims for reimbursement or avoid discrepancies in documentation. Unfortunately, all too often, the skilled therapist speaks one language regarding the resident's progress, while nursing speaks another. Documentation of a resident's function should be consistent and/or any differences should be explained. There may be, for example, documentation from nursing that states a resident is unable to ambulate in his or her room, when that same resident is ambulating with the physical therapist each day with only contact guarding. This kind of discrepancy should be recognized, acknowledged, and explained. Tables 6.11 and 6.12 illustrate examples of nursing documentation that would support the provision of a skilled service, or more accurately describe a resident's performance.

Regardless of whether the nursing restorative care staff, the therapy staff, or a combination of both deliver the rehabilitation, it is vital that all care addresses the resident's goals 24 hours a day. It is incumbent upon all staff members, especially nursing, therapy, and therapeutic recreation, to be familiar with these goals. The entire caregiving staff must work as a team, communicating regularly to ensure that the resident's goals are pursued on all shifts, 7 days a week (see Appendix).

GENERAL DOCUMENTATION AND FOLLOW UP

Accurate and complete documentation—not only on the MDS, as previously discussed, but also in supporting nursing flowsheets and the resident's permanent medical record—is critical for a successful nursing restorative program, to optimize PPS reimbursement, and to prevent fraudulent Medicare/Medicaid claims. It is essential to create a process for capturing essential data on the services provided under nursing restorative care. It is the facility's decision on

TABLE 6.11 Supportive Nursing Documentation for Therapies

Physical Therapy

Functional Skill	Nursing Documentation Example
Bed mobility	• Resident holds onto side rails to pull self onto side. • Two nursing assistants move resident up in bed with use of turning sheet.
Supine to sit → Stand	• Resident can pull self to sitting position with use of side rails. Can swing right leg to floor. Nursing assistant moves left leg to floor. Needs assist of two to lift resident from sitting to standing position. Once standing, can pivot to wheelchair and sit independently.
Transfers	• Transfers from bed to wheelchair with contact assist to cueing of one, to remind resident not to bear weight on left leg. • Requires two to transfer 75% of time, lifting resident from bed to chair. Resident will pivot once lifted to a standing position 25% of time.
Ambulation	• Ambulates 20 feet in hallway with two therapists, one holding gait belt and one following behind with wheelchair. Resident ambulates bent at waist and will sit down without warning. Nursing does not ambulate on unit per therapist recommendation.

Occupational Therapy

Functional Skill	Nursing Documentation Example
Feeding	Feeds self 50% of meal with builtup spoon. Pockets food in right cheek.
Grooming/hygiene	Brushes teeth and combs hair 100% of time if prompted by staff.
Bathing	Needs total assist of one with tub and shower. Washes face and upper body 5% of time.
Dressing	Resident puts on own shirt with setup. For lower body dressing, resident needs total staff assist because he or she is not yet able to use reacher.
Transfer (to toilet, tub)	Transfers to raised toilet seat with assist of one nurse aide for contact guard.
Mobility/wheelchair	Resident propels self from bed to hall (15 feet); forgets to lock breaks 50% of time.
Activity tolerance	Resident complains of fatigue after sitting 1 to 1½ hours in wheelchair.

Nursing Restorative Care Activities

Functional Skill	Nursing Documentation Example
Response to name or voice	Smiles and turns head when greeted 100% of time.
Follow verbal directions	Resident follows simple commands but cannot express needs.
Response to yes or no questions	Nods yes or no correctly 50% of time.
Nonoral communication	Resident is using communications board to request items. When communication board is offered, resident uses it to request items for ADLs. Staff use board to get resident to express needs. Correctly used 80% of time.
Eating	Resident needs to be encouraged to take fluids after three swallows of food. Meal span 30 minutes. Needs to be reminded to tuck chin prior to swallow 4–6 times during each meal.
Orientation	Resident is oriented to place and person, but not time. NOTE: If resident is not oriented, nursing should report how disorientation is interfering with ADLs.

how often to document progress, based on the types of programs offered and the needs of the individual resident. This requirement should be in policy form to ensure compliance and consistent application. Daily completion of the restorative flowsheet (Tables 6.6 and 6.7) will provide the documentation necessary to fulfill the requirement for actual minutes of service provided on a daily basis. Even if the 15 minutes per day required for documentation on the MDS is not met, the use of a daily flow record will ensure timely and accurate documentation of actual services provided. Since these services and the required documentation will be completed by an unlicensed caregiver, family or volunteer, the restorative nurse or licensed

TABLE 6.12 Suggestions for Documenting Resident's Inability to Participate in Therapy

Problem	Solution
Writing that resident simply refused treatment	• Resident unable to participate in therapy today due to not feeling well. • Resident requested that treatment not be provided today because. . . . • Resident requested that therapy be rescheduled when (less fatigued, having less pain, etc.).

Words to avoid	Words to use
Plateauing	Continued steady progress toward goals
Ambulate	Gait training
Maintenance	Continuing treatment plan to include bed mobility, transfer training and progressive training, during the week of.
Patient refuses treatment	Patient unable to participate today due to pain in left lower extremity and primary health care provider informed.
Therapist exercises patient on low mat today.	Patient exercised left lower extremity on low mat and is showing return of muscle tone and mass in left lower extremity.
No change in status	

nurse assigned to that particular resident must routinely review these records to ensure accurate completion and assess the resident's participation in the restorative activity. Often, adjustments to the restorative plan will need to be made, with new goals established and additional interventions incorporated. Although periodic evaluation by the licensed nurse is required, the frequency should reflect the particular needs of the resident. For example, a resident newly discharged from physical therapy who is on a treatment plan of ambulation twice daily for a period of 15 minutes each time to reach a distance of 50 feet may easily reach that goal after a week on a restorative ambulation program and need to have a reassessment and new goal established. Another resident, more physically and mentally challenged with a dressing program of donning and fastening a shirt each morning for 15 minutes, could easily remain at that level for an extended period of time. A restorative policy that allows the licensed nurse discretion to make decisions about the frequency of evaluations would certainly make sense. This would necessitate that licensed staff participating in this process be trained in the assessment process and evaluated regularly for competence. Tables 6.13 and 6.14 illustrate a sample documentation tool that allows for a regular narrative progress note or assessment as well as the use of codes.

Unlicensed caregivers often are more comfortable with coding types of documentation rather than a narrative style. This tool allows the entire interdisciplinary team to have input about the resident's progress. The general rule is that documentation must ensure that the planned restorative nursing services were administered as directed or ordered. The documentation must also contain objective and measurable information so that progress, maintenance, or regression can be recognized from one evaluation to the next. Specific information should also be documented concerning the resident's response to the treatment plan. This would include the amount of assistance required, the device used, the distance, the time required, the progress made, and how well the resident tolerated the activity. This information should be included when describing any restorative activity and needs to be adapted to the particular activity being performed. For example, it is not possible to measure dressing or grooming in terms of distance traveled, but an evaluation of the amount of the activity that was performed with a specific amount of "supervision" or "assistance" is valuable. Restorative documentation may also be included as a part of the generalized nursing documentation if the restorative components are clearly identified. This would most likely necessitate modification of an existing nursing flowsheet to include the specific components required such as minutes spent, resident participation, and response. Most long-term care facilities use a separate restorative documentation system for greater accuracy, ease in monitoring, and consistency in application.

The restorative team will also need to make decisions about assessment procedures and documentation tools to ensure consistency of the data collected. One of the factors that leads to inconsistency is discrepancies in staff performance of functional tests or assessments. The directions and education for performing assessments and using specific tools, should be identified in policies and procedures, and these should be used appropriately and assessed regularly. Although the MDS is a required and necessary assessment tool, it is, as the name describes, a "minimum" assessment, and lacks the specific areas that a restorative care plan must address. For this reason, it is recommended that the restorative team choose an assessment tool or multiple specific tools to identify a

TABLE 6.13   Restorative Care Resident Progress Note

Resident: _____ Room #: _____ Month/Year: _____

☐ Range of motion   ☐ Self-care program/ADLs   ☐Ambulation   ☐ Other _____

☐ _____   ☐ _____   ☐ _____

Ambulatory aids: ☐   Yes   ☐ No

　Type: ☐ Crutches   ☐ Cane(s): __ R   __ L   ☐ Walker   ☐ Other _____

Goal: _____

_____

Plan: ☐ Frequency _____   ☐ Duration _____

Treatment plan:_____

Precautions:_____

Days of the Month

	1	2	3	4	5	6	7	8	9	10	11	12	13	14	15	16
Code/11–7																
Minutes																
Initials																

	17	18	19	20	21	22	23	24	25	26	27	28	29	30	31	
Code/11–7																
Minutes																
Initials																

TABLE 6.14   Restorative Care Resident Progress Notes—Final Documentation

_____

_____

_____

_____

_____

_____

_____

_____

Codes:	5—Met 100% of the goal	R—Refused
	4—Met 80% of the goal	S—Sick
	3—Met 50% of the goal	W—Withheld TX
	2—Met 20% of the goal	Y—Holiday
	1—Met 5% of the goal	D—Discharge
	0—No progress	H—Hospital

resident's needs. There are many tools available that can give accurate measurements and clearly establish a treatment plan. The easiest approach may be to begin with the MDS assessment, together with the facility admission nursing assessment to identify initial restorative needs. For example, if the resident presents with limited range of motion in the right arm and contracture of the right fingers, a more extensive assessment to measure the actual functional loss in these areas would dictate a reasonable goal for the restorative team. Documenting actual degrees of a contracture on an admission assessment provides the opportunity to easily measure progress in terms of additional degrees of motion. Tables 6.15 and 6.16 illustrate the use of a range of motion assessment and initial plan. This assessment tool could be used on admission to establish a treatment plan, then on a quarterly basis to evaluate the plan of care, or when substantial progress or decline is observed. Particularly if a specialized orthotic device is used by the resident, the use of a specific tool would allow measure-

TABLE 6.15   Range of Motion Assessment and Initial Plan: Upper Extremity

1. Inspection:
   a. Alignment
   b. Check skin for color, swelling, masses
   c. Check muscles, and compare both sides for size, symmetry, spasms
   d. Palpate all bones, joints and muscles, for muscle tone, heat, tenderness, swelling, crepitus
2. Check for active and passive range of motion and compare both sides:

Resident's ROM				
Joint	Normal ROM	Right Side	Left Side	Plan
Mouth	• Open and close • Move side to side			
Shoulder	• Shrug shoulders • Flexion 160° • Extension 50°			
Cervical spine	• Extension 55° (backward) • Flexion 45° (forward) • Lateral bending 40° • Rotation 70°			
Thoracic and lumbar spine	• Forward flexion 75° • Hyperextension 30° • Lateral bending 35° rotation			
Elbow	• Flexion 160° • Extension from 160° to 0° • Pronation 90° • Supination 90°			
Hands and wrists	• Metacarpophalangeal hyperextension 30° flexion 90° • Thumb opposition • Forming a fist • Finger adduction and abduction • Wrist flexion 90° and hyperextension 70° • Radial motion 20° • Ulnar motion 55°			
Thumb	• Proximal phalange flexion 70° • Distal phalange flexion 90°			

ment of the progress made and provide direction for change.

When selecting documentation tools or systems of documentation, consider not only the specific needs of the particular resident but also what will capture changes in resident function and be easy for staff to use. If the tools chosen are too complex or time consuming, it will be difficult to maintain compliance with time frames for use. Using the RAI guidelines for completion of the MDS would be a realistic and, in most cases, appropriate reassessment schedule. The RAI requires an initial assessment, followed by reassessments quarterly. These assessments then form the basis for the resident plan of care. Table 6.17 provides an example of a

functional assessment tool to measure a resident's ability to perform a variety of personal care activities. This tool is modeled after the format for completion of the MDS, which requires two separate assessment tasks. Task one is to identify the resident's ability to perform the identified task, using numbers as a code to determine a pattern of independence to dependency. Task two identifies the amount of staff assistance and physical support required. The codes used in this tool match those required by the MDS, and thus staff are already comfortable and competent in judging the appropriate coding documentation.

With the quarterly assessment schedule, the tool easily identifies whether the resident is gaining, los-

TABLE 6.16   Range of Motion Assessment and Initial Plan: Lower Extremity

Joint	Normal ROM	Right Side	Left Side	Plan
Hip	• Flexion (bent knee) 120° • Flexion (straight knee) 90° • Abduction 30°–45° • Adduction 30°–45° • Hyperextension 30° • Internal rotation 40° • External rotation 45°			
Knee	• Flexion 90°–130° • Extension 0°–15°			
Ankle/Feet	• Abduction 10°–20° • Adduction 10°–20° • Dorsiflexion 20° • Plantar flexion 45° • Inversion 30° • Eversion 20°			

Great toe	• Distal phalange flexion 50°
	• Proximal phalange
	    Flexion 35°
	    Extension 80°			

ing, or maintaining function. Also required by documentation standards and regulations for a restorative care program is the licensed nurse signature and date the assessment is performed. Such a tool could be individualized for each resident or used as a standard tool for all residents to measure progress. Reflecting on the areas identified previously for a restorative care program, facility policy should include the use of standardized tools for each of the restorative activities (ROM, splint or brace assistance, bed mobility, ambulation training, transfer training, dressing, grooming, eating or swallowing, amputation or prosthesis train-

ing, and communication training). In general, the federal requirements for restorative care guide the survey teams (and the facility) to expect to find specific documented evidence of these activities, as shown in Table 6.18.

THE RESTORATIVE CARE PLAN

Simply speaking, a care plan is a guide to action. This documented plan enables all members of the interdisciplinary team to understand the goals sought and the

TABLE 6.17   Functional Assessment

Scoring Key for Functional Assessment

1st Column Client's Ability to Perform the Task	2nd Column Amount of Assistance and Physical Staff Support Required
0 = Independent—Requires no staff assistance or supervision. 1 = Supervision—Requires staff supervision, reminders, cueing, and coaching. 2 = Limited Assistance—Requires minimal physical staff assistance during some phase of the activity. 3 = Extensive Assistance—Requires major physical staff assistance to perform activity. 4 = Total Dependent—Requires total physical staff assistance, client unable to perform any part of the activity.	0 = No staff intervention or physical help required. 1 = Staff need to provide setup help to enable client to perform the activity. 2 = The physical assistance of one staff person is needed for the client to perform the activity. 3 = The physical assistance of two or more staff is necessary to do the task.

TABLE 6.18   Federally Required Documentation of Restorative Care Acitivites

1. Document assessment of a resident's physical and mental functional abilities and determination of the resident's needs for staff assistance, assistive devices and/or equipment, and a restorative care program.
2. Document that restorative care and services are being done on a daily basis, or less often if stated on the plan of care.
3. Document that the care plan is being consistently implemented as planned.
4. Document that staff have made aggressive efforts to counsel and offer alternatives to a resident who refuses to participate in care treatment that would maintain or restore functional abilities.
5. Document that decline in a resident's functional abilities was unavoidable.
6. Document that individualized restorative objectives of the plan of care were periodically evaluated and are being met. If objectives are not being met, alternative approaches are documented.
7. Document psychosocial and cognitive deficits that affect a resident's ability to perform activities of daily living, measures instituted to assist a resident to compensate for this loss, and periodic review as to effectiveness of these measures.
8. Document assessment of each resident to see if there are risk factors for falling, development of pressure ulcers, dehydration, and weight loss. If the resident was identified as being at risk for development of any of these problems, there is documented evidence of a prevention plan, how the plan is working, and alternative interventions and results when the plan is not working.
9. Document that residents who are incontinent of bladder receive appropriate treatment and services to prevent urinary tract infection and to restore as much bladder function as possible.
10. Document that residents with a reduction in range of motion have a clinical condition that makes the development of further contractures unavoidable.

TABLE 6.19   Contractures Care Plan

Resident Name: _____   Resident ID#: _____

Date Initiated: _____   Date Resolved: _____

Problem Statement: Contractures r/t: ☐ Immobility   ☐ Decreased mental status

Date	Goals	Approaches/Interventions	Disciplines
	1. Resident will have no further contractures of _____ _____ through the next review date ___ days. 2. Resident will have no increase in contractures of _____ _____ through the next review date: _____ days.	1. ROM w/activities of daily living 2. ROM w/restorative care program _____ _____ 3. Assess resident for new or increase in existing contractures during MDS review. 4. Splint _____ 5. Hand rolls 6. When doing ROM, do not force movement 7. Turn and position every 2 hours. 8. PT/OT evaluation as needed. 9. Use wedges as positioning device for: _____ 10. Encourage resident to move and do ROM of all extremities. 11. Attend exercise program. _____ _____ 12. Special restorative orders: _____ _____ _____ 13. Maintain proper positioning by _____ _____ _____ 14. Medicate for pain prior to ROM.	

TABLE 6.20 Definition and Requirements of the Care Plan

Definition: The care plan is a guide to actions. This documented plan enables all caregivers to understand the goals sought and the specific interventions to achieve those goals.

Requirements
1. Identify the specific activity to be done based on the resident's need.
2. Create measurable goals that are appropriate to the resident's condition with a stated time for reevaluation.
3. List approaches and interventions.
4. State frequency of the activity to be performed.
5. State the duration of the specific activity.
6. Determine who will be responsible and who will deliver the treatment or service.
7. Regularly evaluate the process, and make changes where necessary.

specific interventions identified to achieve those goals. A well-written and understood plan of care can prevent wasted efforts on the part of the team, as well as causative actions that are inappropriate for the individual resident (Table 6.19).

The federal requirement for comprehensive care plans at Section F279 states: "The facility must develop a comprehensive care plan for each resident that includes measurable objectives and timetables to meet a resident's medical, nursing, and mental and psychosocial needs that are identified in the comprehensive assessment" (Health Care Financing Administration, 1999). Developing a restorative care plan is no different that any other resident care plan in that it must contain certain common documentation elements, as described in Table 6.18, and should include the following steps.

Step 1: Identify the Specific Activity To Be Done Based on the Resident's Need

For instance, Mr. S, a resident who presents on a functional assessment with a contracture of the right shoulder, elbow, and wrist due to a stroke will require range-of-motion exercises. Refer to Tables 6.19 and 6.20 for a sample care plan for contractures. It is important to include training and skill practice in the restorative care plan if it will be a part of the activity. The *MDS 2.0*

User's Manual (2002) defines training and skill practice as "activities including repetition, physical or verbal cueing, and task segmentation provided by any staff member or volunteer under the supervision of a licensed nurse."

Step 2: Create Measurable Goals Appropriate to the Resident's Condition With a Stated Time Frame for Reevaluation

There are basically four types of goals that can be considered for each resident. The first is *improvement,* which should be used when a condition can be reversed or when restoration of function can be anticipated. The second is *prevention,* which should be used to prevent complications in a condition or treatment. The third is *palliative,* which is used to provide comfort and support as in an end-stage process. The fourth is *maintenance,* which is used to maintain the current status or level of function and avoid further decline. When stating goals it is important to state a goal for each problem or need identified. These goals must be realistic, practical, and geared to the resident's ability to respond. Goals should always be set *with* the resident, not for the resident. Remember that it is the resident who is trying to meet the goal. Goals may also be identified as short or long term. For restorative care planning, it is often best to identify both the short-term goal and the long-term goal. For example, the long-term goal for the resident with contractures could be that the "resident will achieve 80% of normal function at the end of restorative treatment." However, the short-term goal would better be stated in terms of "the resident will increase range of motion by 5–10 degrees in the next 90 days." In the sample care plan, leave blank spaces between the two stated goals to allow for individualized identification of the areas to be treated and the degree of improvement.

Step 3: List Approaches and Interventions

When selecting care plan approaches, an accurate assessment of the resident's current status as necessary to build on his or her strengths. For instance, if Mr. S (the resident with contractures) is able to participate in active assistive range of motion, then a more accurate, individualized approach would be "active assistive ROM through the restorative care program." Interventions must also reflect current professional standards of practice and facility policy for provision of care. For instance, if the facility does not use hand rolls, but rather a "carrot" device or washcloth for contracture prevention, those terms should be used in the care plan. In general, approaches should be oriented to preserving function and avoiding decline rather than treatment of an existing condition. This focuses on the restorative nature of the approach rather than on the illness or deformity. Most importantly, approaches must incorporate the wishes and abilities of the resident. To use an approach that the resident refuses will only serve to frustrate the resident and the staff. Care plan interventions must, by nature, be developed with the active participation of the resident, significant others, staff, and therapists.

Step 4: Determine the How Often the Activity Is to Be Performed

Ideally, restorative activities are performed on a daily basis or more frequently, as indicated by the needs of the resident and the availability of staff. Documentation for restorative care on the MDS asks for the number of days in the last 7 that the activity has been performed. If your restorative program relies on the availability of only the restorative care aide and not the entire restorative team, it will be difficult to provide activities with any amount of regularity. When considering how often to provide the restorative activity, remember that care may be provided by anyone trained in restorative care. This enables volunteers, family members, therapeutic recreation aides, nursing assistants, and others to provide certain restorative care techniques, under the supervision of the licensed nurse.

Step 5: Determine the Duration of the Activity

Be specific in the care plan about how long the restorative activity should be performed. MDS documentation requires a minimum of 15 minutes per day for each restorative activity; the 15 minutes do not have to occur all at once. Teaching and/or supervising the activity may also be included in the 15 minutes. For instance,

the resident who performs active assistive range of motion together with the nursing assistant twice a day (morning and evening) for 8 minutes each time fulfills the documentation requirement. As an intervention on the care plan, this care could be documented as "active assistive ROM to the right shoulder, elbow, and wrist, for 10 repetitions, twice daily, for 8 minutes each session, with the assistance of the nursing assistant." If this same resident progresses to performing active ROM, the documentation could state, "Active ROM to the right shoulder, elbow, and wrist for 10 repetitions, twice daily for 8 minutes each session, under the supervision of the nursing assistant."

Step 6: Determine Who Will Be Responsible and Who Will Deliver Care

The plan of care for each restorative activity needs to clearly identify who will deliver the treatment and who will be responsible. In the case discussed under step 5 above, it is the nursing assistant. Remember that the requirements for restorative care do not necessarily need to be carried out by nursing staff. The *MDS 2.0 User's Manual* (2002) states, "These activities are carried out or supervised by members of the nursing staff. Sometimes under licensed nurse supervision, other staff and volunteers will be assigned to work with the specific residents." For example, Mr. S has a daughter who visits daily to have supper with her father. She has been trained by the licensed nurse in the techniques involved in the performance of active assistive ROM exercises with her father. As such, she will be included in the restorative plan of care as the person responsible for delivering the ROM exercises in the evening. The appropriate intervention could state, "Active assistive ROM exercises to the right shoulder, wrist, and elbow for 10 repetitions, twice daily, for 8 minutes each session. Daughter to perform activity in the evening."

Step 7: Regularly Evaluate Progress and Make Changes Where Necessary

The nursing process teaches the importance of regular evaluation of the resident plan of care. This is also required for restorative nursing. The *MDS 2.0 User's Manual* (2002) states, "Evidence of periodic evaluation by licensed nurse must be present in the clinical record." Previously in this chapter, the use of a restorative care flow record was discussed, in which the licensed nurse indicates his or her review by signature and/or appropriate comments. This is a regular evaluation that could be performed monthly with the use of each new flow record. The important factor is that the licensed nurse makes the appropriate changes in the plan of care when the evaluation identifies that changes are necessary. The care plan is always what drives the care, and the resident who drives the care plan. So whenever changes in the resident's status indicate changes in a restorative activity, the licensed nurse responsible for that resident is the one who should make those changes. The federal requirements for care plans under CFR 483.20 at section F280 states, "A comprehensive care plan must be developed within 7 days after the completion of the comprehensive assessment; and periodically reviewed and revised by a team of qualified persons after each assessment" (Health Care Financing Administration, 1999).

TABLE 6.21   Essential Components of Care Planning

- There is no right way or only way to write a care plan.
- The care plan is an instrument that is used to communicate clearly.
- Resident assessment is the foundation for a comprehensive care plan.
- The only way to determine a resident's needs is to listen, look, and question.
- The plan must be important for the care and outcome of the resident.
- It must be developed with the active participation of the resident and significant others.
- All caregivers must participate in the development of the care plan.
- Care plans must be working tools for residents, family, and staff.
- It must be understandable to all who use it.
- Keep the care plan simple.
- Keep the care plan current.
- Set goals with the resident rather than for the resident.
- Remember that it is the resident who needs to meet the goals of the plan.
- Believe in the care plan you have developed with the resident, and make it work for him or her.
- Remember the nursing process:
    Assess
    Plan
    Implement
    Evaluate
    Revise

The assessment time frames are also defined in CFR 483.20 as "within 14 days after admission," "within 14 days after the facility determines that there has been a significant change in the resident's physical or mental condition," "not less than once every 12 months," and "not less frequently than once every 3 months."

Most long-term care facilities have an established policy and procedures for completion of the required assessments and care plan process. Restorative nursing plans of care will frequently fit into these time frames and meet the mandatory requirements. However, when the resident's condition requires more frequent assessment and evaluation, it is the responsibility of the licensed nurse to complete this process. Often the resident who has completed an active physical therapy program will require frequent, even daily monitoring by the licensed nurse. The use of daily restorative care flow records will easily record the type and amount of activities performed, but additional documentation will be required in the clinical record to monitor the resident's progress toward any care plan goal. The *Scope and Standards of Gerontological Nursing Practice* (ANA,). at Standard VII, Evaluation, provides excellent guidance: "The nurse continually evaluates the client's and family's responses to interventions in order to determine progress toward goal attainment and to revise the data base, nursing diagnoses, and plan of care." For a summary of this section on the restorative care plan, see Table 6.21.

REIMBURSEMENT FOR RESTORATIVE CARE

For the most part, nursing restorative care is a nursing cost and is not a reimbursable service. However, under the prospective payment system (PPS), facilities can capture costs related to provision of nursing rehabilitation services for a small portion of Medicare residents. Four of the resource utilization groups, or RUGs-III, categories of PPS incorporate the use of nursing rehabilitation/restorative care services. These include rehabilitation low, impaired cognition, behavior problems, and reduced physical function. Of these four RUGs categories, only Rehabilitation Low has a presumption of qualification as skilled care under Part A Medicare. There are relatively few instances when nursing restorative care programs cannot be provided alongside skilled services, either as an extension of those skilled services or as autonomous programs. Collaboration between nursing restorative care and therapy will enhance the care given to residents and ensure Medicare compliance. Most residents whose care is covered by Medicare are appropriate candidates to receive a minimum of two nursing restorative care program activities. Most often, it is recommended that these programs be started as soon after admission as is appropriate. (Watts & Mullins, 2000) Nursing restorative care plays a vital role in the placement of a resident into the rehabilitation low RUGs category. To qualify for this category, there must be at least two nursing restorative activities for 15 or more minutes a day for at least 6 of 7 days, provided in concert with at least 45 minutes of skilled therapy for 3 of 7 days. (Fleishell et al., 2000) Even if a resident has a low weekly need for skilled intervention, the rehab low category usually provides a higher reimbursement rate than most nursing RUGs levels. Examples of this could include the resident with pressure ulcers or positioning issues, or a resident with Parkinson's disease who needs skilled therapy to develop a customized maintenance program. When skilled therapy staff are unable to deliver the required minimum of 5 days of care during the assessment period, a rehab RUGs level (rehab low) can be salvaged if two nursing restorative care activities have been given for 6 days during that assessment period (Watts & Mullins, 2000).

The 7-day assessment time frame is indicated on the MDS as the "observation period" and the specific date is identified in Section A3 of the MDS as the Assessment Reference Date. This is the last day of the MDS observation period, and its purpose is to ensure that all involved staff will be using the same period of time as this assessment period. This assessment date and directions for its use are not new. Under RUGs III and PPS, the Center for Medicare and Medicaid Services (CMS) makes facilities accountable to observe the reference date in order to ensure consistency of the data being collected. It does *not* mean that the assessment has to be recorded on that exact day, as long as the data that is collected, and the questions that are asked, refer to the same block of time. It does mean that assessments cannot be completed and recorded before the end of the assessment period. This assessment reference date is the date from which the reviewer counts back to determine a 7-, 14-, or 30-day observation period, as requested by the MDS.

Although not discussed in this chapter, there are state-specific programs under Medicaid that also will reimburse facilities for restorative care, using the MDS 2.0 as the primary documentation tool. The requirements for reimbursement under Medicaid will generally correlate with those required under PPS; however, the state-specific regulations need to be understood and used to ensure compliance and the accompanying reimbursement.

Payment source should never be a consideration when determining the need for a restorative nursing program or activity. However, knowledge of the conditions for reimbursement under either Medicare or Medicaid will allow a facility to optimize these programs and provide the resident the maximum benefits required by regulation.

The PPS/RUGs III reimbursement system is a complex mixture of categories, minutes of service, and determination of the need for skilled services, and it cannot be fully described in this chapter. What can be attempted is a brief description of each of the Medicare RUGs categories available for reimbursement using restorative care and the criteria that must be achieved.

The first general requirement under each of the reimbursement categories involves the use of two restorative care activities for a minimum of 15 minutes per day of 6 of the last 7 days. Classification for RUGs III is directly affected by these minutes of service provided. Only hands-on restorative care minutes are considered for completing minutes of service. This includes resident time spent in treatment, setup time, and time spent supervising the resident during treatment. It does not include staff time to produce or document treatment. It does not include time spent performing an evaluation. Time spent teaching staff to perform tasks related to the particular restorative care service also does not count as minutes of service. Time spent actually teaching a resident or family caregiver how to perform tasks related to restorative care services for an individual does count as minutes of service when completing the MDS. It is easy to appreciate the importance of using standardized documentation tools to provide supporting data for counting minutes of service. This collected data is reviewed and clarified in determining accuracy of MDS documentation. Nursing assistants and all involved staff will need to be taught specifically how to use the tool so that the information collected is reliable. Repeated intense teaching and additional one-on-one instruction, as indicated, may be necessary to ensure that direct care providers understand expectations and performance parameters.

CMS has additionally qualified that some restorative activities listed on the MDS—when paired together—only count as one restorative activity. This does not preclude staff from providing these two activities concurrently, it only means that, together, the activities will be counted as only one for RUGs III reimbursement. Selecting two or more restorative activities, when done with appropriate residents, helps the residents qualify for the low rehabilitation group, thus optimizing the reimbursement for those activities. The following "pairs" are counted as one:

1. Active/passive ROM: If the resident received passive range of motion (item P3a on the MDS), that counts as one activity. If the resident received active range of motion (item P3b on the MDS), that counts as one activity. If they are both checked, that still counts as one.
2. Bed mobility/walking: If bed mobility (item P3d on the MDS) is checked, it counts as one restorative activity. If walking (item P3f on the MDS) is checked, that counts as one activity. If both are checked, that counts as one.
3. Toileting/bladder retraining: If any scheduled toileting plan (item H3a on the MDS) is checked, that counts as one activity. If bladder retraining is checked (item H3b on the MDS) is checked, that counts as one activity. If they are both checked, it still counts as one.

SPECIFIC RUGS CATEGORIES AFFECTING RESTORATIVE CARE

Rehabilitation Low

This category requires that the resident has received the following during the last 7 days (observation period): (1) 45 or more minutes of skilled rehabilitation therapy; (2) at least 3 days on any combination of the three disciplines (physical therapy, occupational therapy, speech therapy); and (3) two or more nursing restorative services for at least 15 minutes each, with each administered for 6 or more days.

Impaired Cognition

This category requires documentation on the MDS that considers the following factors: (1) coma and not awake and completely dependent in ADLs, (2) short-term memory, (3) daily decision making, (4) making self understood, and (5) eating self-performance. All residents classified into the impaired cognition group are further subdivided on the basis of ADL functioning and nursing rehabilitation.

Behavior

This category requires that the following behaviors have occurred on 4 or more of the last 7 days (as documented on the MDS during that observation period): wandering, physical abuse, verbal abuse, inappropriate behavior, resisting care, hallucinations, and delusions. All residents classified into the behavior group are further subdivided on the basis of ADL functioning and nursing rehabilitation.

Behavior problems often interfere with the resident's ability to cooperate with and stick with a restorative care program. This category adds additional weight in determining the RUGs category an individual falls into, and must be carefully and accurately scored on the MDS under Section E4, Behavior Symptoms. To capture this data, carefully question families, staff, and the resident to obtain an accurate history. In many cases, this MDS section is completed by the social worker. Communication is imperative to collect and document completely and accurately. Flow charts that document specific behaviors may be helpful. You could also provide a list to families, explaining the indicators you need to identify and ask them to circle behavior they see and mark the date and time. The idea is not to encourage recording of symptoms that are not there but to get credit if the resident does exhibit these symptoms. Table 6.22 provides a sample documentation tool used to gather behavioral data during the 7-day observation period.

Reduced Physical Function

Residents who are not classified into one of the above groups (Rehab low, Impaired cognition, Behavior) will fall into the reduced physical function group.

TABLE 6.22 Resident Behavior Data-Gathering Tool

7-Day Observation Period

Resident: _____   Date initiated: _____

Shift: ☐ 7–3   ☐ 3–11   ☐ 11–7

Date: _____

	A	B	A	B	A	B	A	B	A	B	A	B	A	B
	1		2		3		4		5		6		7	
Wandering														
Verbally abusive														
Physically abusive														
Socially inappropriate														
Resists care														

KEY: For each of the following behavioral symptoms listed below, score for A and B.

A = Frequency

0 = Not exhibited

1 = Occurred at least once

2 = Occurred twice

3 = Occurred three times or more

B = Alterability

0 = Behavior not present, or behavior was easily altered

1 = Behavior was not easily altered

These residents will be further subdivided on the basis of ADL functioning and nursing rehabilitation. The criteria for consideration under nursing rehabilitation has been previously discussed in this chapter.

It is important to note that ADLs influence every one of the seven RUGs groups. In order to get credit, the facility must collect objective data for 7 days from all direct care staff on all shifts. This is most accurately done using data-gathering tools, direct observation, and communication. Regardless of whether the nursing restorative care staff, rehabilitation staff, or direct care staff deliver the rehabilitation, it is vital that all care encompasses the resident's goals 24 hours a day. It is incumbent upon all staff members, especially nursing, therapy, and therapeutic recreation, to be familiar with these goals. The entire caregiving team must work as a team, communicating regularly to ensure that the resident's goals are pursued on all shifts, 7 days a week (Watts & Mullins, 2000).

GROUP PROGRAMMING— DOCUMENTATION GUIDE

Group programming is the part of the restorative care program that focuses more on the emotional and social well-being of the individuals while still providing planned opportunities to work on skills, sensory stimulation, exercise, and ambulation. Recreation is a core part of restorative care and has too long been ignored as a therapeutic intervention and tool. Residents moving into long-term care facilities are making emotional, social, and lifestyle adjustments and can receive a great deal of benefit and satisfaction from group restorative activities. Some residents require more encouragement than others, but consistent opportunities to be encouraged and satisfied can go a long way toward helping residents regain control of their lives and feel worthwhile. Every member of the staff is responsible to help residents find ways to bring genuine pleasure into their time. Many disciplines can become involved in group restorative programming. Recreational therapists and recreational aides or activities staff are key in this special programming. Social workers also play a large part in identifying the special interests of residents and making positive suggestions for therapeutic interventions. Maintenance and housekeeping staff can find their own special ways to participate in special programming. All departments (including volunteers and families) are needed for facility-wide projects. Recreational and social activities accompanied by restorative care programs cannot change the disabilities, deficits, and mental status of individuals, but they can provide socialization opportunities that allow older adults to appreciate life and be recognized as individuals with unique qualities.

The purposes and goals of restorative care group programming focus on providing restorative care activities that are fun in a group setting while improving and maintaining the self-esteem of the residents. In addition, these activities should improve motor skills, function, body awareness, cognition, and strength. The group setting provides residents with opportunities to use social graces and express emotions, and it promotes encouragement and recognition among peers.

Structured Classes

Group programming for restorative care must be structured, planned, routinely held, and properly documented. Groups can be planned by the restorative care team, activities staff, or a combination of staff for a truly "team" approach. Scheduled classes or programs may be open for all interested residents to participate, and all residents should be encouraged to attend. Residents with specific restorative care plans that include group activities will be required to participate regularly, with attendance monitored by the staff using the restorative care flowsheet to document minutes of attendance. For attendance at group activities to count toward the restorative care section of the MDS, the number of participants in the class is limited to four residents for each group leader. Group leaders need to be instructed in the goals of the program and each resident's individual plan of restorative care. For example, using Mr. S (the resident identified previously in this chapter who presents on a functional assessment with a contracture of the right shoulder, elbow, and wrist due to a stroke and who requires range of motion), the restorative care team has decided that a group activity situation would increase his ability to participate in restorative care and would enable him to receive encouragement and praise in a group setting for reaching his goals. His care plan will direct his participation in the "Chair Aerobics" class, which is held once a week in the activities room. This class is led by the activities staff for all interested residents. However, to ensure active participation and meet the requirements for group programming for restorative care, the restorative aide will lead four of the residents

in the class who participate in restorative care. This aide has in-depth knowledge of each resident's particular exercise routine and ensures that the interventions in the residents' care plans are met. Mr. S's care plan could state, as an intervention, "Will be an active participant in the chair aerobics class held weekly for 30 minutes. Active range of motion exercises to all upper extremities will be supervised by the restorative aide." Attendance at this group activity could be documented on the MDS as 1 day of the required 6 days of participation in a restorative care activity.

Special attention should be paid to the times and location of group classes to encourage resident participation and staff involvement. Special recognition needs to be given to the participants. Planning group programs is a chance for the staff to let their imaginations run wild and find new and interesting activities that also provide restorative care. Include the residents in the planning. Ask residents what special activities or groups were a vital part of their lives before living in a long-term care setting, and include those ideas in the program, if possible. Some suggestions for restorative care group activities programming can be found in Tables 4.8, 4.9, and 4.10.

OPTIMIZING OPPORTUNITIES

The intent of this chapter on documentation was not only to describe the requirements for accurate and comprehensive documentation of a restorative care program, but also to provide creative ideas for restorative staff to use in program planning and suggestions to optimize precious resources and time. Whether the facility is planning a new restorative care program or seeking ways to improve or expand an existing program, the individual needs of the resident population are what will drive change. First evaluate current provision of restorative type activities (if there is no formal program) or the restorative activities currently provided. Second, evaluate the restorative needs of the residents to determine if these are being met under the present structure. Then ask whether the program is meeting not only the needs of the residents but the documentation and structure requirements for restorative care. The facility will need to clearly identify a few key areas: (1) What residents use what programs? (2) What residents are in need of services that are not currently provided for them? (3) How can restorative activities be paired for each resident to create a therapeutic program that meets the requirements? Some restorative care activities are naturally paired, for example, use of splints and range of motion, transfer skills and scheduled toileting, bed mobility and transfer training, and prosthesis care and ambulation (using the prosthesis). It is not difficult to identify pairs of restorative activities that will benefit the resident as well as meet the documentation requirements of the MDS. Also evaluate existing resources to determine if the program uses them wisely. The following principles can guide existing programs to maximize the use of facilities' primary resource—staff: (1) Clearly define what restorative care activities can be incorporated into the daily care provided by nursing assistants. (2) Provide any necessary education in restorative care activities to direct care staff (be sure to include documentation requirements). (3) Provide documentation tools, education in their use, and easy, structured access to these tools. (4) Provide continued direction and feedback to staff. Then celebrate the rewards—improved resident function, heightened staff motivation, an expanded sense of team, and an increased marketing opportunity.

QUALITY IMPROVEMENT

The restorative program is essential to the facility quality improvement plan, especially as it relates to falls, maintenance of function status, prevention of decline in ADLs, and prevention of contractures. The restorative nurse coordinator's role is to report to the quality improvement committee on the status of the program as a whole and the individuals participating in the program. The role of the restorative nurse coor-

TABLE 6.23 Sample Documentation for Restorative Care Resident Class Attendance

List residents (with room numbers) who are scheduled to attend.
Date: _____

Grooming Tips

_____
_____
_____
_____
_____
_____
_____
_____

TABLE 6.24 Documentation for Ambulation Class Attendance

Park and Dine

_____
_____
_____
_____
_____
_____
_____
_____

TABLE 6.25 Restorative Care Program Quarterly Summary

Indicate the total number of residents participating in the restorative care program.

Program	#	Program	#
Bed mobility		Transfer training	
Ambulation		Range of motion	
Dressing		Grooming	
Splint, cane, braces usage		Communication	
Amputation/prosthesis training		Bladder retraining	
Eating/Swallowing restorative dining		Assistive devices and adaptive equipment	
Scheduled toileting		Other (identify)	

Restorative Care Classes

Class	#	Class	#
Grooming Tips		ADL Fun	
Sensory Stimulation		Range of Motion	
Communication		Isometrics	
Park and Dine		Walk Across America	
Wheelchair Dance		Ballroom Dancing	
Other (Identify)		Other (Identify)	

Number of residents discharged from the program as maximum benefit: _____

Number of residents admitted to the program since last summary: _____

Coordinator Signature: _____ Date: _____

dinator is critical to the success of the restorative care program, and is necessary under the PPS reimbursement requirements. Many long-term care facilities include the restorative nurse coordinator responsibilities in the job description of a management-level licensed nurse, such as charge nurse, unit manager, or assistant director. This is especially indicated in small organizations whose resident population does not support a separate restorative nurse coordinator position. This position requires independent function, and adequate time needs to be allotted to perform the variety of duties. Good interpersonal skills and the ability to lead a diverse team are essential traits. It is the Restorative Nurse Coordinator who "owns" the program, coaches and teaches the staff, and keeps everyone motivated and working collectively as a team. The use of summary tools and lists of participants should be a part of the documentation duties of the restorative nurse coordinator. This will simplify organization of the program and make reporting easier, more effective, and accurate. Good reporting mechanisms will also validate the effectiveness of the program and prove positive resident outcomes. The particular needs of the residents and the structure of the program will dictate the specific tools needed to enhance the organization of the program and meet the requirements of the quality improvement program. Tables 6.23, 6.24, and 6.25 are samples of the type of documentation that should be kept current and reported regularly.

Quality is an attitude that accepts nothing less than the agreed-upon standard in product or service. In the long-term care setting, staff must strive for quality in the services they provide and must also do everything possible to assist residents in attaining quality in all aspects of their lives. Achieving quality, or excellence, is a multidimensional and ongoing process that takes great commitment from an organization's leaders. With any aspect of a well-organized quality improvement program, all areas of care delivery should be monitored to ensure that residents receive optimal care opportunities or actual delivery of that care. This is also true of the restorative care program. Any and all aspects of the program may need to be critically evaluated through the quality improvement process to ensure that the goals and objectives of the program are being met, especially as they relate to improved resident care and outcomes.

As with any quality improvement activity, monitoring of the restorative care program is an ongoing and active process, with identified tools, plans, and reports. The goal of this process is two-fold: (1) to ensure that each resident receives the care identified in his or her individual restorative care plan and (2) to ensure that each aspect of the program has followed the identified program objectives, policies, and procedures. Some type of quality improvement activity should be performed on a monthly basis, and a resultant action plan should be developed for any identified problems. Choose a variety of methods to monitor different restorative activities, and alternate the areas monitored to ensure that all aspects of the program are evaluated. Below are suggestions for quality improvement restorative areas to monitor.

Quality Indicators

Quality indicators are measurements that relate to the quality of care given. These measurements are calculated using the assessment data imported from the MDS data entry system. The quality indicator is often a combination of items identified from documentation on individual items from the MDS. Table 6.26 identifies the 11 quality indicator domains and also the 24 quality indicators. What is important to note is that the quality indicators are only the starting point of evaluating the quality of care. They do not determine compliance or noncompliance with regulations or quality standards. Since the quality indicators are directly derived from MDS data, their accuracy depends on accurate completion of the MDS. Facilities can easily access their quality indicator reports using the MDS transmission route system and following menu options to quality improvement reports.

With the advent of quality indicators driving a focused survey process, facilities now have an additional impetus to implement effective nursing restorative care systems. Two quality indicator domains directly relate to restorative care, elimination/continence and physical functioning. Restorative care programs can positively influence indicators of decline in late loss ADLs, prevalence of weight loss, prevalence of dehydration, prevalence of tube feeding, and incidence of decline in range of motion. Many other domains and quality indicators also indirectly relate to restorative activities. These can include prevalence of falls, bowel or bladder incontinence, prevalence of daily physical restraints, prevalence of bedbound residents, and prevalence of pressure ulcers, among others. Table

TABLE 6.26   MDS Quality Indicators

Domain	Quality Indicator	Type of Indicator
Accidents	Incident of new fractures	Outcome
	Prevalence of falls	Outcome
Behavioral/emotional patterns	Prevalence of behavioral symptoms affecting others	Outcome
	Prevalence of symptoms of depression	Outcome
	Prevalence of depression with no antidepressant therapy	Both
Clinical management	Use of nine or more different medications	Process
Cognitive patterns	Onset of cognitive impairment	Outcome
Elimination continence	Prevalence of bladder or bowel incontinence	Outcome
	Prevalence of occasional or frequent bladder or bowel incontinence without a toileting plan	Both
	Prevalence of indwelling catheters	Process
	Prevalence of fecal impaction	Outcome
Infection control	Prevalence of urinary tract infections	Outcome
Nutrition	Prevalence of weight loss	Outcome
	Prevalence of tube feeding	Process
	Prevalence of dehydration	Outcome
Physical functioning	Prevalence of bedbound residents	Outcome
	Incidence of decline in late-loss ADLs	Outcome
	Incidence of decline in ROM	Outcome
Psychotropic drug use	Prevalence of antipsychotic use in the absence of psychotic and related conditions	Process
	Prevalence of antianxiety/hypnotic use	Process
	Prevalence of hypnotic use more than two times in last week	Process
Quality of life	Prevalence of daily physical restraints	Process
	Prevalence of little or no activity	Outcome
Skin care	Prevalence of stage 1–4 pressure ulcers	Outcome

6.27 provides a visual grid of the clinical links among MDS-based quality indicator domains and quality indicators. The restorative care coordinator should always review these quality indicator reports on a monthly basis to determine any problematic areas or any decline in the facility's percentile ranking among other like facilities, and to monitor the status of individual residents.

Review of Restorative Program Monthly Summary

Careful evaluation, on a monthly basis, of residents' progress in the restorative care program would certainly qualify as a quality improvement activity. This review might include the following questions: (1) Are residents making progress toward established goals? (2) Are new residents assessed and placed on the program? (3) Are residents achieving maximum benefit? (4) Are too many residents dropped from the program due to lack of participation? (5) Are all the developed programs being used regularly? (6) Do all caregivers and staff participate in the program?

Review of Individual Residents and Programs

A primary objective of the restorative care program is to restore or maintain residents at their maximum potential. Review of a random sample of residents participating in the restorative care program is a good method for evaluating the effectiveness of the program. Any aspect of the restorative care program may be monitored as part of a regular quality improvement program. For instance, to determine whether turning and position activities are being performed on a specific unit as per the resident plan of care, a simple process would be to select residents on the unit and

TABLE 6.27 Clinical Links Among MDS-Based Quality Indicator Domains and Quality Indicators

Accidents	Behavior/Emotional Patterns	Clinical Management—Use of 9+ Medications
New fracture	Use of 9+ medications	Falls
Falls	Incidence of cognitive impairment	Symptoms of depression
Use of 9+ medications	Fecal impaction	Incidence of cognitive impairment
Weight loss	Urinary tract infection	Bowel/bladder incontinence
Dehydration	Weight loss	Fecal impaction
Decline in late-loss ADLs	Dehydration	Weight loss
Psychotropic drug use (any)	Bedbound residents	Dehydration
Daily physical restraints	Psychotropic drug use (any)	Decline in late-loss ADLs
	Daily physical restraints	Psychotropic drug use (any)
	Little or no activities	

Cognitive Patterns—Incidence of Cognitive Impairment	Elimination/Incontinence	Infection Control–Urinary Tract Infections
Behavior affecting others	Use of 9+ medications	Behavior affecting others
Symptoms of depression	Urinary tract infections	Use of 9+ medications
Fecal impaction	Dehydration	Incidence of cognitive impairment
Urinary tract infections	Bedfast residents	Bowel/bladder incontinence
Weight loss	Decline in late-loss ADLs	Indwelling catheter
Dehydration	Psychotropic drug use (any)	Dehydration
Decline in late-loss ADLs	Daily physical restraints	Bedbound residents
Psychotropic drug use (any)	Pressure sores	Pressure sores
Daily physical restraints		
Little or no activities		

Nutrition/Eating	Physical Functioning	Psychotropic Drug Use
Symptoms of depression	New fracture	Falls
Use of 9+ medications	Falls	Behavior affecting others
Incidence of cognitive impairment	Symptoms of depression	Symptoms of depression
Fecal impaction	Use of 9+ medications	Use of 9+ medications
Urinary tract infections	Incidence of cognitive impairment	Incidence of cognitive impairment
Bedbound residents	Bowel/bladder incontinence	Bowel/bladder incontinence
Decline in late-loss ADLs	Urinary tract infections	Weight loss
Psychotropic drug use	Weight loss	Decline in late-loss ADLs
Daily physical restraints	Dehydration	Daily physical restraints
Pressure sores	Psychotropic drug use	Little or no activities
	Daily physical restraints	
	Little or no activities	
	Pressure sores	

Quality Of Life	Skin Care
Falls (physical restraints)	New fractures
Behavior affecting others	Bowel/bladder incontinence
Symptoms of depression	Indwelling catheters
Weight loss (restraints)	Weight loss
Dehydration (restraints)	Dehydration
Bedbound	Bedbound residents
Decline in late-loss ADLs	Daily physical restraints
Decline in rom (restraints)	
Psychotropic drug use	
Pressure sores	
Restraints	

monitor for evidence that the activity is being performed. This type of audit activity could be performed on a variety of restorative care program activities and reported as often as deemed necessary.

The baseline assessment tools recommended in chapter 3 (Table 3.2) provide a useful way to follow individual residents over time and establish changes. The Barthel Index, for example, can help to document changes in residents (e.g., from needing two people to help with transfers to being able to transfer with assistance of one person). While these tools require some additional staff time to complete, the information obtained would certainly facilitate the nurse's ability to complete or to provide information for completion of required assessment tools such and the MDS and the OASIS, which are not as able to pick up small functional status changes. There are no clear guidelines about when follow-up assessments should be made, and therefore assessment frequency should be established based on facility need. In the long-term care setting, follow up can easily coincide with MDS evaluation time. Other options are to evaluate routinely every 6 months, or annually. When changes are recognized, the restorative care plan may need to be revised to better fit the needs of the resident.

SUMMARY

This chapter discusses the regulations related to restorative care activities and the impact of those regulations on documentation of services and reimbursement of restorative care. It is vital to maintain accurate and complete documentation of restorative care in the resident's medical record, including specific sections of the MDS and a comprehensive restorative care plan. Further, nursing flowsheets, assessment tools, and progress notes must describe restorative interventions and identify caregivers. Thorough documentation of nursing restorative care programs through quality improvement activities also demonstrates the facility's commitment to improvement or maintenance of resident function. Training for all restorative care providers, including nurses, nursing assistants, non-nursing staff, volunteers, and family members, must also be documented and available for review as part of the restorative care program. A well-managed, effective, and accurately documented restorative care program is the key to maintaining compliance with regulations and ensuring positive resident outcomes.

REFERENCES

American Health Care Association. (1999). *The long term care survey.*

American Nurses' Association, Council on Gerontological Nursing, Executive Committee. (1995). *Scope and standards of gerontological nursing practice.* Washington, DC: American Nurses Association.

Center for Medicare and Medicaid Services. (1995). *Long term care facility resident assessment instrument (RAI) user's manual.*

———. (2000). *Minimum data set (MDS)—Version 2.0.*

Collard, B.J. (1998). *Restorative nursing revisited, regulatory readiness.* Briggs Corporation.

Code of Maryland Regulations. (1998). Department of Health and Mental Hygiene, 10.07.02 Comprehensive Care Facilities and Extended Care Facilities

Fleishell, A., Mullins, D., & Watts, P. (2000). Introduction to nursing rehabilitation/restorative care. *Advance for Nurses, 2*(21),

Health Care Financing Administration. (April 10, 2000). *Federal Register*

Health Care Financing Administration. (1999). Medicare and Medicaid Requirements for Long Term Care Facilities Regulations, 42 CFR Part 483, Subpart B.

Fleishell, A., & Resnick, B. (2001). *Stayin' alive—The restorative care manual.* Joanne Wilson's Gerontological Nursing Ventures.

MDS 2.0 user's manual, revised. (2002). Briggs Corporation.

Omnibus Budget Reconciliation Act OBRA 1987 OBRA Guidelines www.vericare.com/OBRA.htm

Watts, P., & Mullins, D. (2000). Skilled therapy & nursing rehabilitation—Either, neither or both? *Advance for Nurses,*

APPENDIX

The Interdisciplinary Team Approach

Marjorie Simpson

INTRODUCTION

Generally, restorative care activities are performed by nurses and nursing assistants, since these individuals provide the majority of the hands-on caregiving. Although the majority of the responsibility for developing, implementing, and monitoring a restorative care program falls to the nursing department, an interdisciplinary approach to restorative care enhances patient outcomes and the overall quality of the care that is provided to older adults. An interdisciplinary team approach involves collaborative communication and shared goals and responsibilities among professionals and paraprofessionals involved in the care of the older individual. In addition to health care providers in nursing, rehabilitation, primary health care (physicians and advanced practice nurses), social workers, and activities, the older adults' family and others such as housekeepers, maintenance workers, or waitresses/hostesses should be included in restorative care training and performance of restorative care activities. These individuals, as appropriate, should be involved in setting goals, planning, and executing the restorative care program. Each discipline brings a unique perspective to the team and helps to ensure that all of the older individuals' physical, psychological, and cognitive needs are met. Care plan meetings and restorative care rounds that include all of the disciplines are an effective way to facilitate communication and collaboration. This chapter briefly reviews interdisciplinary teamwork.

GERIATRIC TEAMS

Interdisciplinary teams are important in providing care for older adults, but interdisciplinary teamwork is rarely a teaching focus. Health care professionals are commonly left to develop teamwork skills by chance. Health care team function differs from traditional group theory in that all members of the team are caregivers. A noncompetitive, supportive atmosphere is most appropriate for patient care. The primary group task is to maximize patient functional independence and personal goals. Leadership is task dependent.

In 1997, the Hartford Institute supported the development of eight geriatric interdisciplinary training teams (GITT) at eight different academic medical centers in the United States. The teams demonstrated different ways of educating interdisciplinary teams and helping these teams to effectively communicate to improve care to older adults (Long & Wilson, 2001; Williams, Remington, & Foulk, 2002). The GITT programs have developed numerous tools to help developing teams evaluate team process, such as the Team Fitness Test (Table A.1) and the Team Observation Tool (Table A.2). In addition, the GITT programs have developed invaluable resources that can be used to facilitate communication among teams and help develop appropriate and effective team interactions (Geriatric Interdisciplinary Team Training, 2003). Effective team process is essential to all aspects of geriatric care, and is central to restorative care services and programs. All members of the team have important and equal roles in developing and implementing restorative care services to older individuals, and in implementing a restorative care philosophy of care. First and foremost, it is important to establish that all team members agree and support this type of philosophy of care, and that all are committed to encouraging older adults to participate in functional activities at their highest level of function.

TABLE A.1   Team Fitness Test

Rate each of the following statements as it applies to your team, using the following rating scale:

This statement *definitely applies to our team.*	4
This statement applies to our team *most of the time.*	3
This statement is *occasionally* true for our team.	2
This statement *does not describe* our team at all.	1

Enter the score you believe appropriate for each statement beside the statement number on the Scoring Sheet.

_____ 1. Each team member has an equal voice.

_____ 2. Members make team meetings a priority.

_____ 3. Team members know they can depend on one another.

_____ 4. Our mandate, goals, and objectives are clear and agreed upon.

_____ 5. Team members fulfill their commitments.

_____ 6. Team members see participation as a responsibility.

_____ 7. Our meetings produce excellent outcomes.

_____ 8. There is a feeling of openness and trust in our team.

_____ 9. We have strong, agreed-upon beliefs about how to achieve success.

_____ 10. Each team member demonstrates a sense of shared responsibility for the success of the team.

_____ 11. Input from team members is used whenever possible.

_____ 12. We all participate fully in team meetings.

_____ 13. Team members do not allow personal priorities/agendas to hinder team effectiveness.

_____ 14. Our roles are clearly defined and accepted as defined by all team members.

_____ 15. Team members keep each other well informed.

_____ 16. We involve the right people in decisions.

_____ 17. In team meetings we stay on track and on time.

_____ 18. Team members feel free to give their honest opinions.

_____ 19. If we were asked to list team priorities, our lists would be very similar.

_____ 20. Team members take initiative to put forth ideas and concerns.

_____ 21. Team members are kept well informed.

_____ 22. We are skilled in reaching consensus.

_____ 23. Team members respect each other.

_____ 24. When making decisions, we agree on priorities.

_____ 25. Each team member pulls his or her own weight.

CARE PLAN MEETINGS AND RESTORATIVE CARE ROUNDS

Long-term care facilities are required to have routine interdisciplinary care plan meetings to discuss resident care and establish goals and interventions to ensure that residents' highest level of physical and psychological functioning is attained and maintained. In some states, assisted living facilities have similar requirements that care planning sessions must occur (Assisted Living Workgroup, 2003). In the home setting, care

TABLE A.2   Team Observation Tool

Team:_____   Date:_____

Team Goals

1. Does this team have an apparent goal? __Yes __No What is it? _____
_____

Professional Roles

2. Circle the disciplines attending the meeting.   MD MSW NP RN Pharm OT PT

3. Do team members appear knowledgeable about their roles? _Y _N

4. Do team members appear knowledgeable about the roles of other disciplines? _Y _N

5. Are there disciplines participating on the team whose roles you are not familiar with? _Y _N
If so, which ones?
_____

Leadership

6. Who is (are) the team leader(s)?_____

7. Does the leadership change during the meeting? _Y _N

8. What behaviors do the leaders use (summarizing, initiating . . .)
_____
_____

Communication and Conflict

9. Is there any open sharing of information? _Y _N

10. Note any barriers to communication you observe (side conversations...)_____
_____

11. Is there an opportunity for differences of options to be discussed? _Y _N

12. What are the examples of conflict? How were they handled?

Conflict	Strategies Used to Handle

Meeting Skills

13. How is the meeting organized? (agenda . . .) _____
_____

Outcome

14. What was accomplished or produced during the meeting?_____
_____

15. Are decisions and next steps clear? _Y _N

16. Was the meeting efficient? _Y _N Elaborate _____
_____

Source: D. Long and N. Wilson (Eds.)

planning may be done face-to-face with a limited number of health care team members. Others, however, may be involved intermittently. Care plan meetings are an ideal format for reviewing restorative care goals and approaches to meeting goals. When an older adult is identified as having a problem with mobility or self-care, a restorative care plan that addresses the problem should be established and included in the resident's care plan. Interdisciplinary discussion offers each discipline the opportunity to have input into establishing goals and approaches to meet those goals. In addition, interdisciplinary collaboration provides a means of ensuring that all of the disciplines are aware of what each is contributing to promote functioning. For example, the nursing staff may not realize that an older adult enjoys attending a group exercise activity that is conducted three times a week by the activities department. Through group collaboration, the nursing

staff may alter the schedule for activities of daily living or dressing changes to facilitate time for the individual to participate in the exercise class.

Restorative care rounds can be conducted in a meeting style format with group discussion, or they can be conducted as actual rounds where the team walks through the facility and visualizes residents as they conduct self-care, mobility, or feeding activities. For those in the home setting, virtual team meetings and collaboration can occur via Internet interactions or conference calls. Meetings can be held before or after routine care plan meetings where each discipline has an opportunity to present an older adult who may benefit from restorative care or who requires a change in short- or long-term goals or the approaches implemented to meet the goals. Walking team rounds have the added benefit of the entire team being able to visualize residents during their routine activities. Semi-for-

TABLE A.3 Interdisciplinary Roles in Restorative Care Programs

Discipline	Direct Care of Older Adults	Restorative Care Role
Nursing assistants	Assist with mobility and activities of daily living, including bathing, dressing, grooming, and feeding	Provide the majority of the restorative care activities
Nursing	Assess and monitor residents' medical conditions and response to pharmacologic and nonpharmacologic treatments	Evaluate for the ability to participate in restorative care activities; establish short-term and long-term goals with input from other members of the team; ongoing evaluation of goal achievement
Primary health care providers (physicians, advanced practice nurses, physician's assistant)	Conduct history and physical; diagnose and treat illnesses and injuries; order and interpret diagnostic tests; prescribe medications in most states	Conduct prescreening for restorative care; treat illnesses and injuries that are inhibiting an individual from participating in restorative care activities
Physical therapists	Treat self-care and mobility deficits with exercise and other treatments	Refer residents to restorative care; instruct staff in mobility techniques and assistive devices; serve as consultant to other disciplines
Occupational therapists	Treat self-care deficits with therapeutic activities; train in the use of adaptive devices	Refer residents to restorative care; instruct staff in use of adaptive devices; serve as consultant to other disciplines
Speech-language pathologists	Treat speech, swallowing, and cognitive disorders with therapeutic activities and exercises	Refer residents to restorative care; instruct staff in speech, swallowing, and cognitive techniques and assistive devices; serve as consultant to other disciplines
Activities staff	Coordinate and conduct group exercise and activity classes	Encourage participation in exercise classes and walking groups
Social work	Assist residents in obtaining services; conduct counseling and psychotherapy	Work with individuals to obtain Medicaid or other insurance to cover adaptive equipment; conduct counseling with residents with emotional problems that are interfering with participation in restorative care activities
Ancillary staff	Work in dietary, housekeeping, laundry, maintenance, and admissions	Help motivate residents to participate in restorative care activities; with training, assist with feeding, walking, and exercise programs

mal and formal evaluations with the input of the team can be conducted immediately. With both formats, the appropriate follow up should be established for each individual who was discussed. For example, Mrs. G's son feels that she is having difficulty eating and chewing her food, and the social worker reports this to the interdisciplinary team during restorative care rounds. The group then identifies the need for a mechanically altered diet and a speech therapist evaluation. The nurse obtains orders for both from the facility's nurse practitioner, and the speech therapist conducts the evaluation to identify the need for swallowing exercises or adaptive equipment.

SUMMARY

Restorative care programs are established, executed, and monitored by nursing; however, many different disciplines and individuals play key roles in the success of a restorative care program (Table A.3). Primary health care providers screen older individuals for restorative care activities and treat any medical conditions that result in symptoms that limit their functioning, such as pain and shortness of breath. Collaboration between the rehabilitation staff and the nursing staff can promote referrals for rehabilitation to help individuals attain their highest level of functioning. After an individual is discharged from rehabilitation, nursing staff can establish restorative care activities and goals to help the individual maintain his or her highest level of functioning. Activities staff and other ancillary staff can be trained to conduct restorative care activities such as group exercise, walking, and restorative feeding. Social workers can assist residents and family members in psychological issues that may interfere with motivation and participating with restorative care activities. Using an interdisciplinary team approach for a restorative care program results in the different disciplines involved in resident care establishing and working toward mutual goals.

REFERENCES

Assisted Living Workgroup. (2003). *Recommendations to the Senate Subcommittee on Aging.* Retrieved August 2003 from http://www.aahsa.org/alw.htm

Geriatric Interdisciplinary Team Training. Retrieved August 2003, from http://www.gitt.org/files/creating_the_GITT_Team.doc

Long, D., & Wilson, N. (Eds). (2001). *Houston GITT curriculum.* Houston, TX: Baylor College of Medicine Huffington Center on Aging.

U.S. Department of Labor, Bureau of Labor Statistics. (2002). *Nursing, psychiatric, and home health aides.* Retrieved June 20, 2003, from http://www.bls.gov/oco/text/ocos165.txt

Vincent, K.R., Vincent, H.K., Braith, R.W., Lennon, S.L., & Lowenthal, D.T. (2002). Resistance exercise training attenuates exercise-induced lipid peroxidation in the elderly. *European Journal of Applied Physiology, 87*(4–5), 416–423.

Williams, B.C., Remington, T., & Foulk, M. (2002). Teaching interdisciplinary geriatrics team care. Academic Medicine, 77(9), 935.

Index

Active range of motion, 115
Activities of daily living
  component parts of, 75
  as defined by federal regulations,
    113
  definition of, 56
Activity tolerance, 121
ADLS, components of, 76
Aerobic exercise, 71
Affective states, 7
Age–associated changes, 98
Aggression, 63
Aging, physiological changes
  associated with, 98
Agitation, 62, 63
Alzheimer's groups, 91
Ambulation, 79, 121
  class attendance, documentation
    for, 134
  definition of, 79
  groups, recommendations for, 90
Ambulatory older adults, exercise
  program for, 87–90
Amputation, 115
Antalgic gait, 69
Antalgic gonalgic gait, 69
Anterior cerebral artery, 61
Anxiety, 63
Appetite, changes in, 63
Arteries, decreased compliance of, 98
Assistance with tasks, 75–76
Atrophy, 98

Barriers to implementation of
  restorative care, 8–9
Barthel Index, 136
  definition of, 56
Bathing, 83, 121

Bed mobility, 115, 121
Bedbound, exercise program for,
  87–90
Behavioral Pathology Scale, 63
Beliefs, 97
Beta–adrenergic stimulation,
  decreased response to, 98
Bicycling, 71
Bladder retraining programs,
  definition of activities under,
  118
Blood flow, decreased, 98
Brain, 98
Break down of tasks, 75–76
Breathing exercises, pursed lip, 108
Brief Psychiatric Rating Scale, 63

Calcification, of valves, 98
Cardiac index, decreased, 98
Cardiac output, decreased, 98
Cardiovascular review, in older
  adults, 58
Cardiovascular system, physical
  examination of, 64–65
Care plan
  definition, 127
  requirements of, 127
Care planning, essential components
  of, 129
Caregiver behavior checklist, 83
  use of, 83
Caregivers, education of, 17–45
Caregiving staff barriers, 8
Carotid artery, 61
Case examples to facilitate discussion
  during week one inservice
  training, 41

Cautious gait, 69
Cell proliferation, function, decrease
  in, 98
Cerebellar ataxic gait, 69
Chair aerobics, 91
Champion
  of goal, 50
  involved in ongoing evaluation, 50
  role in motivation of staff
    education, 48–50
  use of cues, 49
Champion concept, 16
Checklist for restorative care
  evaluation, 55
Chronic illness, impact on motivation,
  99–100
Class attendance
  documentation for, 134
  documentation for restorative care
    resident, 134
Clock drawing scoring, 70
Coding, Minimum Data Set
  documentation, 118–119
Cognition
  in older adults, 62–64
  physical examination of, 67–70
Cognitive impairment!
  group classes for those with, 91
  independent function, strategies to
    promote, 104
  motivation issues in, 104
Cognitive measurement tools, 63
Cognitive patterns, 136
Cohen–Mansfield Agitation Index, 63
COMAR 10.07.02.12s, 113
Communication, 115
Constipation, 63
  complications of, 58

Continence, Minimum Data Set, 118
Contractures, 67
   care plan, 126
Cost, as barrier to adherence, 16
Cues to encourage restorative care
    activities, 49–50

Deconditioning, checklist for
    evidence of, 107
Delirium, 62
   characteristics of, 62
Delusions, 131
Dementia, 62
   characteristics of, 62

Dementia–related gait, 69
Depression, 62, 63, 101
   characteristics of, 62
   with cognitive disorders, 101–102
   typical, atypical signs of, 63
Designation of restorative care, 3–4
Digestive secretion enzymes, 98
Dining environment, modifications
    of, 80
Disability Assessment for Dementia,
   63
Documentation, 112–138
   in education of caregivers, 44
   federally required, 126
Dressing, 84–85, 115, 121
   independence, how to achieve, 84

Eating, 80–82, 115, 121
Education
   of caregivers, 17–45
   effect on behavior, 17
Emotional patterns, 137
Enabling environment, 74–75
Enactive mastery experience, 7
Encouragement, verbal, 105
Environment, motivational impact of,
    103–104
   assisted living, 103
   home setting, 103–104
Evaluation of older adults, 53–73
   affective states, 62–64
   cardiovascular review, 58
   cognition, 62–64
   gastrointestinal review, 58–59
   genitourinary review, 59–60
   integumentary review, 62
   musculoskeletal review, 60–62
   neurological review, 60–62

physical exam, 64–70
   affective states, 67–70
   cardiovascular system, 64–65
   cognition, 67–70
   gastrointestinal system, 65
   genitourinary system, 65–66
   head, 64
   integumentary system, 70
   musculoskeletal system, 66
   neurological system, 66–68
   respiratory system, 65
   respiratory review, 58
   screening for exercise activities,
    71–72
   sensory changes, 58
   site–specific evaluation tools,
    70–71
   taking history, 53–57
   functional assessment, 56–57
   medications, 54
   nutritional history, 56
   past medical history, 54
   past surgical history, 54–55
   social history, 55–56
Exercise, 71, 86
   benefits of, 86
   definitions, 71
   as fun, 108–109
   program, 87–90
   screening for, 71–72
   warning signs to recognize during,
    72

Falls, 60
   evaluation of, 61
Fatigue, 63
   interventions to manage, 108
Fear, 97, 106
   interventions to decrease,
    107–108
Federal requirements, 112–113
Federally required documentation,
   126
Feeding, 121
Feeding assistance
   assessment, 80
   modifications of, 80
   quality of, 81–82
Festinating gait, 69
Final documentation, restorative care
    resident progress notes, 123
Flexibility, decreased, 98
Follow verbal directions, 121

Food service, modifications of, 80
Frontal lobe gait, 69
Functional assessment, 56–57, 125
   staging, 63
Functional incontinence, 59
Functional performance, older adults,
    1–2
Functional skills, 77–86, 121

Gait, 66
   disorders of, 69
Gardening, 71
Gastrointestinal review, in older
    adults, 58–59
General activities, definition of, 77
General documentation, follow up,
    120–125
Genitourinary review, in older adults,
    59–60
Genitourinary system, physical
    examination of, 65–66
Geriatric Depression Scale, 63
Getting hurt, fear of, interventions to
    decrease, 107–108
Glial cells, changes in, 98
Global Deterioration Scale, 63
Goals
   attainment scales, 75
   challenge, proximity, 50
   identification, 97
   of restorative care, 3
   specificity, 50
Gonalgic gait, 69
Grooming, 83–84, 121
Group classes
   for those with cognitive
    impairment, 91
   well–attended, recommendations
    for, 91
Group programming documentation
    guide, 132–133
   structured classes, 132–133
Guidelines for development of goals,
   50
Guilt, 63

Hallucinations, 131
Hamilton Anxiety Inventory, 63
Hamilton Depression Inventory, 63
Head, physical examination of, 64
Hearing
   changes, 99
   disorders, 99

interventions to augment, 99
Heart, 98
Helplessness, feelings of, 63
"Highest practicable," determination of, 112
History taking, of older adults, 53–57
  functional assessment, 56–57
  medications, 54
  nutritional history, 56
  past medical history, 54
  past surgical history, 54–55
  social history, 55–56
Home health care!, 9
  Outcome and Assessment Information Set, 70
Hostility, 63
Hyperkineticity, 62
Hypertension, increased, 98
Hypoperfusion, 98

Identification of goals, influence of, 96
Immune system, 98
Impaired cognition, 131
Implementation of Balanced Budget Act, 114
Improving self–grooming skills, effect of, 83
Inability to bathe, effects of, 83
Inability to participate in therapy, documenting, 122
Inadequate staffing, 16
Inconsistency, factors leading to, 123
Incontinence, type of, 59
Incorporation exercise into daily activities, 42
Incorporation of restorative care activities, in education of caregivers, 44–45
Independent function, cognitively impaired older adults, strategies to promote, 104
Individual state regulations, supersede federal statutes, 113
Individualized care, 97
Infection control, 136
Inservice education, powerpoint presentations for, 18–40
Instrumental activities of daily living, 57
  definition of, 56

Integumentary review, in older adults, 62
Integumentary system, physical examination of, 70
Internal Carotid artery, 61
Interventions to influence nursing assistant behavior, 74
Isometric exercise, 71

Job performance, restorative care philosophy, staff education, 13–52
Joint pain, 63

Katz Index of ADLS, 56
  definition of, 56
Kidney function, 98
Kinesthetic sense, changes in, 99

Lack of motivation to continue intervention, 16
Lack of perceived benefit, as barrier to adherence, 16
Leadership role, in philosophy of restorative care implementation, 6
Level of self–esteem, 15
List of functional scales, 56
List of weekly classes for 6–week training program, 17
Locomotion, 79
  definition of, 79
Long–term, short–term goals, nursing assistant approaches, examples of, 49
Lower extremity, range of motion assessment, 125
Lung, 98
  volume, decreased, 98

Manual muscle testing, steps for doing, 68
Marks Sheehan Phobia Scale, 63
MDS. See Minimum Data Set
Medications
  in history taking, 54
  impact on motivation, 100–101
Memory changes, 63
Methods to ensure restorative care success, 43
Middle cerebral artery, 61
Minimal long–term benefits, 16
Mini–mental state examination, 69

Minimum Data Set, 48, 70
  assessment reference date, definition of, 129
  continence, 118
  documentation
  coding, 118–119
  nursing rehabilitation/restorative coding, 118–119
  long–term care sites, 70
  for providers of restorative care services, 114–118
  quality indicator, domains, quality indicators, clinical links, 137
  quality indicators, 136
  requirements for documentation, assessment, 113
  resident assessment documentation requirements, 113
  User's Manual, definition of functional activities, 115
  version 2.0, special treatment, procedures, 114
Minimum Data Set 2.9, user's manual, 128
Mobility, 77–78
Mobility/wheelchair, 121
Moderate exercise, 71
Mood, impact on motivation, 101–102
Motivation, 96–111
  age changes related to, 96–99
  in education of caregivers, 43–44
  interventions to improve, 97
  loss of, 63
  of staff, 13–52
  affective states, 46–47
  champion's role, 48–50
  cues to encourage restorative care activities, 49–50
  education of caregivers, 17–45
  documentation, 44
  incorporation of restorative care activities, 44–45
  motivation, 43–44
  restorative care activities, 41–42
  restorative care intervention, 42–43
  syllabus for, 41–45
  enactive attainment, 47–48
  older adults, evaluating, 48
  philosophy of restorative care and, 13–52
  progress evaluation, 50

Motivation *(continued)*
    restorative care philosophy, 13–52
    restorative care plan, developing,
        49
    self–efficacy
      benefit of, 16–17
      outcome expectations,
            strengthening, 45–48
    self–efficacy approach, 16
    self–esteem and job performance,
        15
    training interventions, 15–16
    verbal persuasion, 45–46
    vicarious experiences, 46
Motivational interventions, to
        augment function, 104–109
Motivational poster, 105
Muscle strength, tool to record, 68
Muscle strength grading, 67
Musculoskeletal review, in older
        adults, 60–62
Musculoskeletal system, physical
        examination of, 66

Name, voice, response to, 121
Neurological system, physical
        examination of, 66–68
Neurons, glial cells, changes in, 98
Nonambulatory, and ambulatory older
        adults, exercise program for,
        87–90
Nonoral communication, 121
Nursing assistant restorative care
        activities, components of, 16
Nursing assistants, training
        interventions, 7–8, 78
Nursing rehabilitation/restorative
        coding, for Minimum Data Set
        documentation, 118–119
Nursing restorative care activities,
        121
Nutrition, 136
Nutritional history, 56

OBRA. See Omnibus Budget
        Reconciliation Act
Observation period, resident behavior
        data–gathering tool, 132
Obsessive–compulsive disorder, 63
Occupational therapy, 121
Older adults
    evaluation, 53–73
    cardiovascular review, 58

cognition, 62–64
gastrointestinal review, 58–59
genitourinary review, 59–60
integumentary review, 62
musculoskeletal review, 60–62
physical exam, 64–70
    cardiovascular system, 64–65
    cognition, 67–70
    gastrointestinal system, 65
    genitourinary system, 65–66
    head, 64
    integumentary system, 70
    musculoskeletal system, 66
    neurological system, 66–68
    respiratory system, 65
respiratory review, 58
screening for exercise activities,
        71–72
sensory changes, 58
site–specific evaluation tools,
        70–71
functional performance of, 1–2
screening for exercise activities,
        71–72
site–specific evaluation tools,
        70–71
Omnibus Budget Reconciliation Act,
        5
guidelines, mandate, 6
MDS. See Minimum Data Set
requirements for, 113–114
Minimum Data Set, requirements
        for, 113–114
skilled nursing facilities and, 112
Opportunities, optimizing, 133–134
Orientation, 121
Origin of restorative care, 2–3
Outcome and assessment information
        set, 9
Overflow incontinence, 59
Overview of education program for
        restorative care, 10

Pain, 97, 106
    assessment, 107
    checklist, 106
    interventions to decrease, 107
Parkinsonian gait, 69
Parkinson's disease, 61
    signs and symptoms of, 61
Past medical history, 54
Past surgical history, 54–55
Patient history, components of, 53

Performance goals, 74
Peripheral vestibular imbalance, 69
Pessimism, 63
Philosophy of restorative care, 4–5
    staff education, motivation, 13–52
Physical activity, 71
Physical exam, older adults, 64–70
    cardiovascular system, 64–65
    cognition, 67–70
    gastrointestinal system, 65
    genitourinary system, 65–66
    head, 64
    integumentary system, 70
    musculoskeletal system, 66
    neurological system, 66–68
    respiratory system, 65
Physical therapy, 121
Physiological changes, associated
        with aging, 98
Podalgic gait, 69
Poor pay, 16
Positive and Negative Syndrome
        Scale, 63
Posterior cerebral, artery, 61
Practice, importance of, 76
Pre–employment
        telemarketing–training
        program, effect on
        self–efficacy, 7
Prescreening of older adults, for safe
        exercise, need for, 71
Prior research on restorative care,
        5–6
Process of restorative care, 74–76.
        See Restorative care
Progress note, restorative care
        resident, 122
Progressive Deterioration Scale, 63
Prosthesis care, 115
Psychological problems associated
        with aging, 62–64
Psychosis, behavior, 63
Psychotropic drug use, 136
Pursed lip breathing exercises, 108

Quality improvement, 134–138
    individual residents, review of,
        136–138
    monthly summary, for review of
        restorative program, 135–136
    programs, review of, 136–138
    quality indicators, 135
Quality indicator, 136

Quality of feeding assistance
  assessment, 81–82
Quality of life, 136
Quarterly summary, restorative care
  program, 134

Range of motion, 115
  exercises, 78
  lower extremity, 125
  upper extremity, 124
Recognition
  insufficient, as barrier to adherence,
    16
  use of, 109–110
Reduced physical function, 131–132
Regulations for long–term care
  facilities, 112–114
Rehabilitation, 131
  defined, 2
  focus on, 119
Rehabilitation nursing
  defined, 2
  goal of, 2
Reimbursement, for restorative care,
  112–138
Reinforcement, use of, 109–110
Remaining abilities, strengths, 74
Repetition, 76
Resident Assessment Instrument,
  User's Manual, 114
Resident behavior data–gathering
  tool, observation period, 132
Resistive exercise, 71
Respiratory review, in older adults, 58
Respiratory system, physical
  examination of, 65
Restorative care
  activities of, 74–95
  affective states, 46–47
  ambulation, 79
  assistance, 75–76
  barriers to implementation of, 8–9
  bathing, 83
  break down of tasks, 75–76
  champion's role, 48–50
  cues to encourage restorative care
    activities, 49–50
  definitive of, 2–3
  designation of, 3–4
  documentation, 112–138
  dressing, 84–85
  eating, 80–82
  education of caregivers, 17–45

documentation, 44
incorporation of restorative care
  activities, 44–45
motivation, 43–44
restorative care activities, 41–42
restorative care intervention, 42–43
syllabus for, 41–45
in education of caregivers, 41–42
enabling environment, 74–75
enactive attainment, 47–48
evaluating older adult for, 53–73
exercise, 86
flowsheet, 116–117
functional skills, performance of,
  77–86
goals of, 3
grooming, 83–84
implementation of philosophy, 6
integrated programs, 4
intervention, in education of
  caregivers, 42–43
interventions to influence nursing
  assistant behavior, 74
job performance, 15
locomotion, 79
mobility, 77–78
motivation of older adult, 96–111
nursing, components of, 113
nursing assistant behavior, training
  interventions influencing, 78
older adults, evaluating, 48
Omnibus Budget Reconciliation
  Act guidelines mandate, 6
origin of, 2–3
overview of, 1–12
philosophy, 13–52
staff education, 13–52
philosophy of, 13–52
plan, 125–129
practice, 76
prior research, 5–6
process of restorative care, 74–76
progress evaluation, 50
rehabilitation, 119
reimbursement, 112–138
remaining abilities, strengths, 74
repetition, 76
resident progress notes, 122
final documentation, 123
restorative care plan, developing,
  49
self–care skills, 77
self–efficacy, 6–7, 16

benefit of, 16–17
outcome expectations,
  strengthening, 45–48
self–esteem, 15
settings, application in, 9–10
staff education, motivation,
  philosophy, 13–52
toileting, 85–86
training interventions, 6, 7–8,
  15–16
transfer techniques, 78–79
verbal persuasion, 45–46
vicarious experiences, 46
Restorative nursing focus on, 119
Rewards
  goals as, 50
  use of, 109–110
Role models, exposure to, 102
Running, 71

Screening for exercise activities,
  71–72
Self–care skills, 77
Self–determination, 97
Self–efficacy framework, 7, 15
  in training, 6–7
Self–esteem, decreased, 63
Self–feeding, 80
Self–modeling, 109
Self–toileting, importance of, 85
Sensations, unpleasant, identifying,
  106
Sensory ataxic gait, 69
Sensory changes, in older adults, 58
Services to older adult, goal of, 9
Shortness of breath, 106
  interventions to decrease sensations
    of, 108
Site–specific evaluation tools, in
  examination of older adults,
  70–71
Skilled therapy, nursing restorative
  care services, 119
Skin, 98
  care of, 136
Sleep
  disorders, 62–64
  patterns, changes in, 63
  sleep cycle, age–related changes in,
    63
Social history, 55–56
Social support, 97
Social withdrawal, 63

Somatic complaints, 63
Spastic gait, 69
Spastic paraparesis, 69
Spirituality, 97
Splint or brace assistance, 115
Staff education, 17–45
   champion's role, 48–50
   documentation, 44
   incorporation of restorative care
      activities, 44–45
   motivation, 13–52
   affective states, 46–47
   champion's role, 48–50
   cues to encourage restorative care
      activities, 49–50
   education of caregivers, 17–45
    documentation, 44
    incorporation of restorative care
      activities, 44–45
    motivation, 43–44
    restorative care activities, 41–42
    restorative care intervention,
      42–43
    syllabus for, 41–45
   enactive attainment, 47–48
   older adults, evaluating, 48
   progress evaluation, 50
   restorative care philosophy, 13–52
   restorative care plan, developing,
      49
   self–efficacy
    benefit of, 16–17
    outcome expectations,
      strengthening, 45–48
   self–efficacy approach, 16
   self–esteem and job performance,
      15
   training interventions, 15–16
   verbal persuasion, 45–46
   vicarious experiences, 46
   restorative care activities, 41–42

restorative care intervention,
   42–43
  syllabus for, 41–45
Staff turnover, 16
Stairwalking, 71
Steppage gait, 69
Stomach, 98
Stress incontinence, 59
Stroke, 61
  signs, symptoms of, 61
Supine to site–stand, 121
Syllabus, in education of caregivers,
   41–45
System of least prompts, definition of,
   76
Systolic hypertension, increased, 98

Tasks, break down of, 75–76
Task–specific activities, definition of,
   77
Telemarketing–training program,
   pre–employment, effect on
   self–efficacy, 7
Therapies, nursing documentation
   examples for, 121
Three Rs, 109–110
Toileting, 85–86
  definition of activities under
    scheduled, 118
  independence, importance of,
    85–86
Training interventions
  to influence behavior of nursing
    assistants, 7–8
Transfer techniques, 78–79

Unpleasant sensations, 97
  decreasing, 106–107
  identifying, 106
Upper extremity, range of motion
   assessment, 124

Urge incontinence, 59
Urinary incontinence, 59

Vascular system, 98
  changes in, 98
Ventricles, decreased compliance of,
   98
Verbal abuse, 131
Verbal encouragement, 104–106
Verbal persuasion, 7
Vertebrobasilar system, 61
Vertigo, 61
Vestibular ataxic gait, 69
Vicarious experience, physiological,
   affective states, 7
Vision, interventions to improve, 99
Visual changes, 98–99
Voice, response to, 121

Waddling gait, 69
Walking, 71, 115
Walking groups, recommendations
   for, 90
Wandering, 131
Warning signs, to recognize during
   exercise, 72
Washing windows, 71
Well–attended group classes,
   recommendations for, 91
Wheel of motivation, 96–97
Wheelchair, acceleration mobility
   dependence, 79
Wheelchair dancing, 91
Wheeling self, 71
Workload, as barrier to adherence,
   16

Yale Depression Screening Tool, 70
Yale–Brown Obsessive Compulsive
   Scale, 63